RESTORATION

Seven Promises of God

Barbara A. Perkins, M.A.

Foreword by
Iyanla Vanzant

KP Publishing Company

Copyright 2020 by Barbara A. Perkins, M.A.

All rights reserved. In accordance with the U.S. Copyright Act of 1976, the scanning, uploading, and electronic sharing of any part of this book without the permission of the publisher is unlawful piracy and theft of the author's intellectual property. If you would like to use material from this book (other than for review purposes), prior written permission must be obtained by contacting the publisher at books@knowledgepowerinc.com.

Thank you for your support of the author's rights.

ISBN: 978-1-950936-18-2 (Hardcover)
ISBN: 978-1-950936-19-9 (Paperback)
ISBN: 978-1-950936-20-5 (E-Book)
Library of Congress Control Number: 2019911986

Edited by: Stacie Fujii
Proofreader: Delerice Mackey
Cover Art: Dr. Synthia Saint James
Cover Design: Juan Roberts, Creative Lunacy
Interior Designer: Creative Lunacy
Literary Director: Sandra L. Slayton

THE HOLY BIBLE, NEW INTERNATIONAL VERSION® NIV®
Copyright © 1973, 1978, 1984 by International Bible Society®
Used by permission. All rights reserved worldwide.

Published by:

KP Publishing Company

Other Books By

BARBARA A. PERKINS, M.A.

**The Magic of Mentoring:
Pearls of Wisdom — Second Edition**

The Coaching Series:

Seven Little Books on Coaching Yourself
Marriage

Seven Little Books on Coaching Yourself
Grief

Seven Little Books on Coaching Yourself
Betrayal

Coming Soon:

Seven Little Books on Coaching Yourself
Entrepreneurship

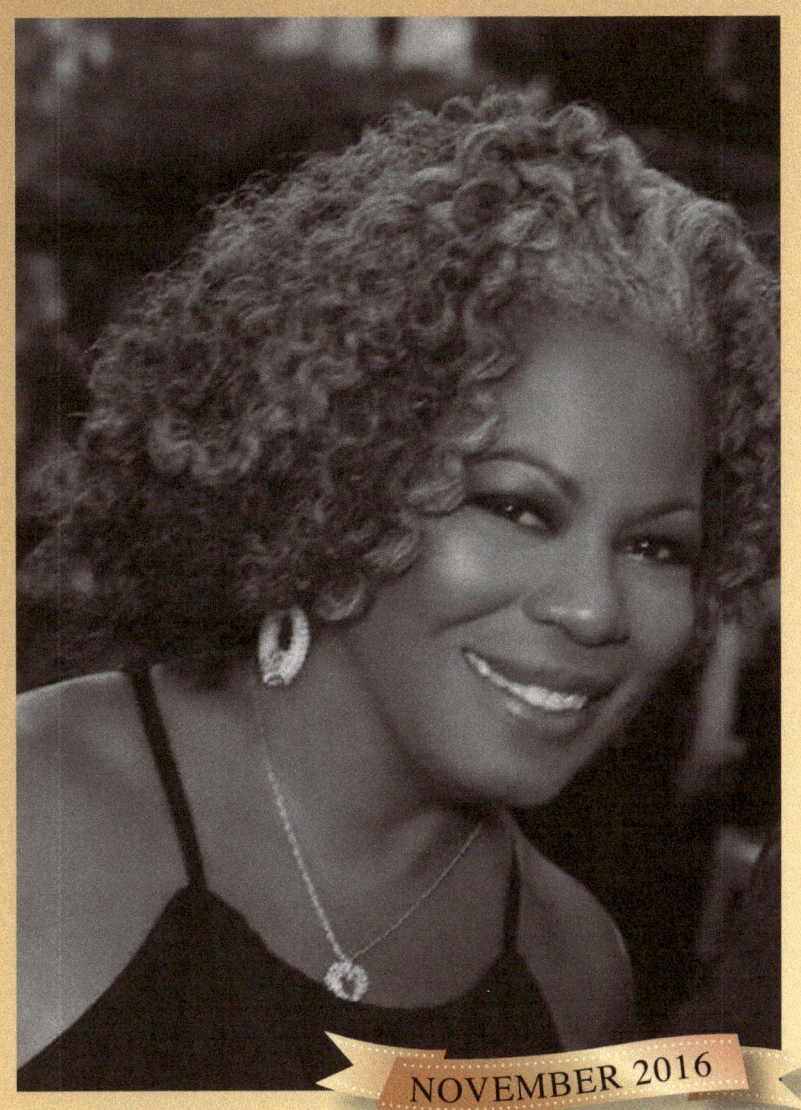
NOVEMBER 2016

DEDICATION

To Stanley Perkins, my beloved husband and friend for 34 years, I dedicate this book to you for who you are as a husband, father, friend and caregiver extraordinaire. This new road you are walking with me, hand in hand, with love and enormous patience, is my greatest blessing.

To Debra C. Thompson, it is difficult to find the words to express my love for you. I am eternally grateful to our mother for the gift of you as a big sister and best friend. Just the thought of being here at this moment in time, without you, overwhelms me. Making it through the first months of this journey would have been so different had you not been here to take the lead as you did. I love you sister and trust you like no other.

To Kelsey and Cody, you are my greatest inspirations. You bring me joy and I am most proud to be your mother. Continue loving each other, checking for each other and being available to each other no matter what happens in this life.

To my baby Emir Stanley Harrison, nothing could have prepared me for the fountain of love for you that flows inside of me. God knew I needed to be present for your arrival. He knew that my life here would be complete once I had a chance to offer and experience "grandmother" love. I vow to introduce you to the God who shepherded you into our lives and who will lead you for the rest of your life.

FOREWORD

Receiving by text, the news of the diagnoses given to Barbara, gave me time and the opportunity to be still and pray before calling her as she had asked in her text. This road was all too familiar to me. I knew the common emotions that often take center stage in the minds of far too many women, when confronted with this information. My responsibility as a spiritual teacher and faith walker is to disrupt any notion of fear, defeat or worse.

My first question to my beloved was, "what are you thinking?" I did not take it for granted that I was among the few she would speak her deepest fears, thoughts, questions and concerns. My response was, "This cancer is not yours. Can you hear and accept that?"

I never believed that this cancer was meant to take up permanent residence in Barbara's body. I sensed restoration from the very beginning. A few weeks later, when she told me about writing this book, I was not a bit surprised. A book that would detail a journey to complete healing and bear witness to the unmatched power of prayer, we can never have too many.

Restoration: Seven Promises of God, paints a vivid picture of courage. Barbara shares her faith and exposes her vulnerabilities. Through her experience she gives voice to others who may be unable to articulate the raging range of emotions that become the unwelcomed guest when faced with such an unpleasant situation. Prepare yourself to read about the painful truth of cancer. You will read about the thief that cancer is and how its sole purpose is to steal your life and take away any joy you have. I trust that you will be as grateful as I am to be a witness to this victory story told with grace.

IYANLA VANZANT

RESTORATION
Seven Promises of God

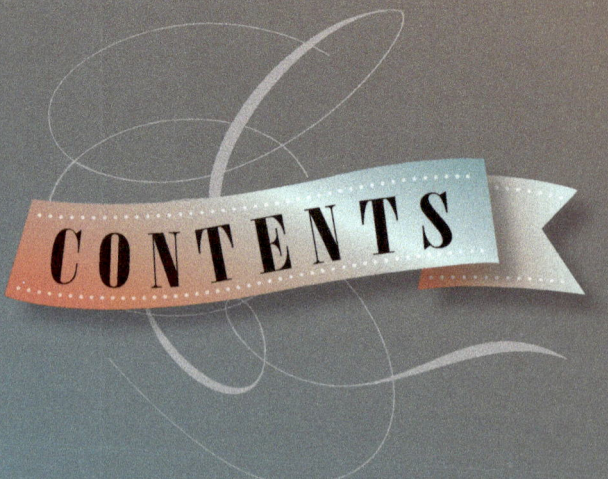

Dedication	x
Foreword	xii
Introduction	xvii
Chapter 1: Restoration	1
Chapter 2: Unleashing the Power of Prayer	27
Chapter 3: Transformation	53
Chapter 4: Forgive and Forget	81
Chapter 5: Divine Assignment	99
Chapter 6: Blessed to be a Blessing	117
Chapter 7: Whole, Perfect, and Complete	137
Colossal Thank You	163
About the Author	167
Acknowledgments	170
"Your Gift" Healing Prayer Gift	175

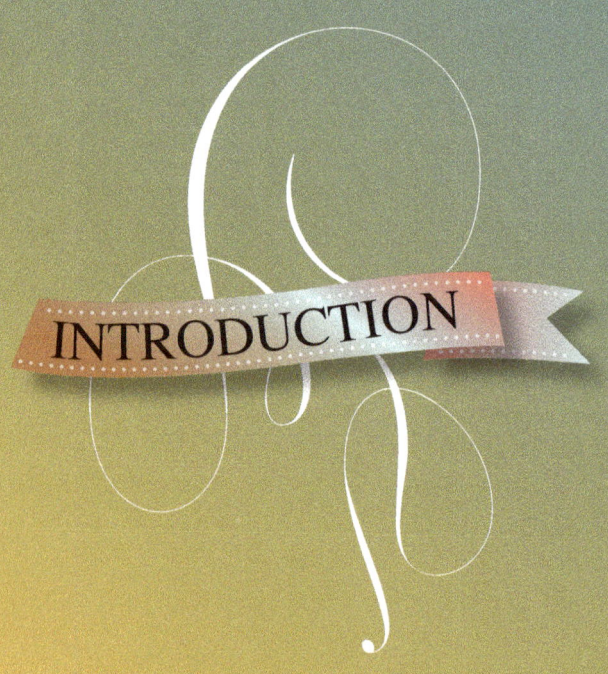
INTRODUCTION

December 9, 2016, I received the call from Dr. Renee Cotter, my gynecologist for almost 20 years, informing me of the results from the biopsy taken from my right breast and lymph nodes under my right arm. "I am sorry Barbara . . . the results show you have an aggressive form of invasive ductal carcinoma with lymph nodes involvement. It is important that you find an oncologist right away and a surgeon." It all went blank from there. I do not remember how the conversation ended, but somewhere in the closing I heard, "take good care of yourself."

I was petrified walking into my first visit to Dr. Amy Law's office two weeks after getting the results of the biopsies. Stanley and I held hands walking in as my sister Debra and daughter, Kelsey, walked behind us. I had not really cried yet because Stanley was so broken up and emotional. I felt I had to be strong for him. When I entered the beautiful building named the Eisenhower Lucy Curci Cancer Center, it all became real in that moment. The tears swelled up in my eyes, my breathing became labored and I could not get my thoughts together. Questions flooded my mind, one right after another. These questions were not for Dr. Law, they were for God.

I found Dr. Law to be detailed, extremely patient and very personable. She answered almost every question Debra, Kelsey and I thought of before we had a chance to ask. She physically wrote her own notes for us on three pages from a legal-size pad. She explained that she preferred if we just listened and not try to take notes. During that visit, Dr. Law measured the two tumors, which seemed to have grown bigger in just two weeks. She told us that one tumor was about 4 centimeters and the other much smaller. She also told us that she thought the cancer was most likely stage II but was concerned about the fast pace at which the tumors were growing. She expressed concern that the cancer had reached the lymph nodes.

The following week, I had an MRI, and a Positron Emission Tomography (PET) scan, which allowed the doctors to check for diseases throughout my body, using a radioactive tracer. Just days following these procedures, I was scheduled to begin four rounds of chemotherapy through a medical port that would be surgically implanted in my chest.

On January 6, the date of my first chemotherapy treatment, Dr. Law measured the two tumors again, and found they had grown, one to almost 6 centimeters. The other one was too deep into the tissue to measure, but it was smaller. She confirmed the cancer was stage III and far more aggressive than she thought before. I was now ready for my talk with God.

The only way I can describe my first treatment is that it was a wipe out. Not even giving birth to my children could compare to the emotional and physical impact that chemo had on me. Holding a thought in my head for any length of time seemed impossible. Being able to explain to my husband and sister how I felt was impossible. This was the first time I could remember that my words simply failed me. My prayers were in short simple questions, statements and requests. "Help me God. What should I do God? I know you are not going to leave me now, God?" It was easier to allow others to pray for me than for me to pray for myself.

I realized that I was in total fear of facing God. Guilt had gripped and pinned me down with brute force. I wondered had I brought this cancer on myself and now my entire family would suffer? It did not help that a few "well-meaning" friends called to chastise me for spending so much of my time helping others over the years, and now, here I stood in need of help. I did not understand what they meant. The implication was that I did not take care of myself to the degree that I tried to help others and therefore I allowed cancer to come into my body.

Two of these calls genuinely unnerved me. They caused me to shut down and turn my telephone over to Debra to screen all calls.

Surprisingly, it would take days before I could finally have a talk with God. Yes, I had prayed, but I lacked the courage to have the real conversation. I sought help from a trusted spiritual leader. She helped me with thinking about how to open myself to God and to wait for an answer. She reminded me how to be still and listen to God's specific words. She reminded me of the secret place where God had visited me before, during past life events that were too big for me to handle by myself.

For years I had worked as a life coach and successfully helped hundreds of people work through life-changing events. Yet, somehow, I had no idea how to coach myself in these first weeks. Remaining calm under pressure was routine for me. I was trained in the late 1970's as a flight attendant and have lived with a 36-year veteran of the fire department for 34 years.

But with this diagnosis there was a major storm brewing under my physical surface. I could feel the break down getting ready to happen.

It happened as I was preparing for my daily 6:30 am prayer call with a group of intergenerational women I have been praying with for three years. Right there in Genesis 9:13-17, I was reminded of God's covenant.

> "I have placed my bow in the clouds; it will be the symbol of the covenant between me and the earth. When I bring clouds over the earth and the bow appears in the clouds, I will remember the covenant between me and you and every living being among all the creatures. Floodwaters will never again destroy all creatures. The bow will be in the clouds, and upon seeing it I will remember the enduring covenant between God and every living being of all the earth's creatures." God said to Noah, "This is the symbol of the covenant that I have set up between me and all creatures on earth."

I read that and remembered a few years back, my dear sister-friend, internationally known fine artist, Dr. Synthia Saint James shared with me a painting she did of a fire rainbow. I had never heard of such a thing, but it was unusual, and intriguing. Then later that same morning, as I was taking my walk in our quiet neighborhood in Rancho Mirage, California, looking straight ahead of me, right above the Santa Rosa Mountains, a rainbow with the most vibrant colors appeared. I heard in my spirit the word RESTORED.

The tears running down my face for the duration of my walk illustrated the profoundly intimate conversation I was having with God. There were so many things I had tucked away, in the crevices of myself. I knew there were secrets I had kept hidden even from God I thought. Over the years I continued stuffing things in spaces with the intention of coming back and cleaning them up, but never did. Now, here I was, staring these mishaps and violations of my faith dead in the face. My body, mind and spirit were laden with grief and despair. Dis-ease had turned into disease and came to attack me in the most vulnerable of places: my breast.

On this walk, with the rainbow before me, I confessed out loud many of the things for which I wanted forgiveness. I proclaimed what I believed about God, who is the only grantor of unwavering grace and mercy. I admitted out loud that I was afraid. I shouted to God that I did not want to be separated from Him under any circumstances. It seemed like every one of *Aristotle's List of Emotions* had taken over me at once. Fear, pity, anger, jealousy, contempt, love, and confidence, seven of the strongest emotions, all paid me a visit on this one-mile walk.

For each emotion, a scripture came to my mind and I could respond. Seven times this happened, and at the end of my walk I prayed: "Dear God, thank you for your promise to restore me your daughter, Barbara Ann Perkins. Thank you for the seven promises and your covenant with me. Thank you God for putting a bow in the sky, a fire rainbow, to remind me of your covenant."

It was during that prayer that I received the title of this book: *Restoration: Seven Promises of God*.

I called Synthia immediately to share this idea of writing this book. I discussed my vision for the cover of the book. Dr. Saint James' paintings have covered over 80 published works, including Terry McMillian's *Waiting to Exhale* and Iyanla Vanzant's *Acts of Faith*. I knew this book had to have the burst of color and majestic feeling that is uniquely present in Synthia's work. She was so happy that I called her to share this idea. She had been praying for me daily on her morning beach walk and sending me beautiful messages of hope and inspiration. We discussed the book and the message I felt led to share within these pages. We discussed the cover briefly. Within a few weeks, my vision was transferred by one of the most creative people in the world and came to life on her canvas.

A day or two after talking with Synthia, I shared the idea with Debra, who I thought would say, "great sister, but not now." I thought for a moment my sister would feel like I was taking on too difficult of a project, as I often do. Debra, lives in Fort Lauderdale, Florida with her husband Bruce. She is my oldest sister and first of 10 siblings. Debra and Bruce were at my side only two days after being diagnosed. We had all planned to be together for the Christmas holidays. She stayed for a total of six months, going home for only a few weeks in between my treatments.

I thought for sure she would put her foot down and not agree to my taking on the task of writing a book during my treatments. To my surprise, Debra was elated to see my passion and hear all about the message this book would have. She joined me immediately on my faith walk, even with the promise of my suffering from "chemo brain" (memory loss due to chemo) and believed that I could write this story.

The number seven is a significant number to this project. It is a number that has significant spiritual meaning. Seven is used 735 times in the Bible. It is used 54 times in Revelations. Jesus performed seven miracles on the Sabbath. It is the number of completion and perfection.

In this book there are seven chapters, with seven specific women included that serve as witnesses of God's fulfilling promises. All are survivors of something major in life. A few are spiritual practitioners, while others are teachers of the gospel of Jesus Christ. They are Reverend Lori Billingsley, Reverend Beverly Biddle, survivor Kathlyn Adams-Seay, survivor Tshombe Buckman, survivor Tia Morris, survivor Tammilee Jules, and survivor Julia Cooksey. Their stories and lessons lifted and empowered me at times when the writing was not easy.

I also share lessons from one of the first families I met when I arrived in Los Angeles in 1984. Dwan and Nate Fortier are survivors and their story continues to encourage me daily. Prepare to be shaken by some of the stories. I did not hold anything back. There were some difficult choices I had to make during this journey. There were times when my spirit was badly bruised, and it had nothing to do with the medication. I had to learn how to listen, but not hear some of the feedback and unsolicited advice given to me by some who thought they were being helpful. Friendships strained and friendships rekindled are all a part of the healing process. To God be the glory, I made it through.

My desire for you as you read this book is that you receive the confirmation of your own restoration. I pray that your rainbow will show up as mine did, and that there is an exclamation point at the end. At the end of each chapter, I offer you a space for your personal expressions, thoughts or questions. There is also a reminder of one of God's promises to us. I trust you will find the reflection pages to be what you need to begin your new road towards your own healing and restoration. I pray God's blessings over your life. I pray for your peace of mind and healthy body.

"But I will restore you to health and heal your wounds, declares the LORD . . ."

JEREMIAH 30:17

CHAPTER 1
RESTORATION

There were so many thoughts racing through my head on the morning of my first visit to Dr. Karl A. Schulz's office. Dr. Schulz, a noted and widely sought-after surgeon from the Eisenhower Medical Center in Rancho Mirage, California, came highly recommended by other patients. Ironically, he was also the unanimous choice of my three best friends: Kathy, Cynthia, and Cheryl. They had all committed themselves to researching, contacting and selecting the best person for the job, and all roads led to Dr. Schulz.

It had been two weeks since I had received the life altering, devastating test results. I had not figured out what I was going to ask of God. I had not fully accepted the news and was still thinking that my diagnosis was a gigantic mistake. This was not a conversation I could have with my two young adult children. *How was I going to get myself out of this? Come on fearless Barbara Ann, the young girl who was always chosen for the big jobs in elementary school and in children's church while growing up in The Bahamas. What is the next move?* These were my thoughts and questions to myself.

I remember thinking, maybe even praying, that it could not be as bad as the doctors wanted me to believe it was. I think I tried to make a deal with God very early on, quietly asking Him to allow some type of test results mix up to be found, so that this would all be sorted out and life would resume. Of course, in my resuming of life, I would be much more aware of just how fragile life is and be more attentive to the most important things in my life. I also reminded God in those first few weeks that while He knew my strength and how much I could handle; He knew my weaknesses. He knew about the things I tried to hide from myself. He knew that I had almost cracked under the pressure of having to explain why I decided to walk away from a perfectly good marriage in my early twenties. He knew the guilt I felt about hurting such a kind man and disappointing those who had high hopes for us.

I reminded God of the years of work I had to do on myself to become the confident woman presented to the world today. He knew me when I felt trapped in feelings of being unworthy, fearful and not enough. Surely, God would not want me to slip back into my not so distant past. Please God, make it something different from cancer because this might just be too much for even me.

The list of questions my big sister, Debra, and I had for Dr. Schulz was not unusually long for families in this same situation. Of course, on top of the list was the question everyone seemed to want to know: What was my stage? We soon learned. It was a few days before I realized Dr. Schulz had not answered that question directly. "The cancer is invasive and very aggressive Mrs. Perkins. The results of the biopsies show a second tumor that is smaller and behind the larger tumor. Also, there is lymph node involvement. We don't know how many lymph nodes at this time, but after you see Dr. Law, your oncologist, we will discuss an aggressive treatment plan. You are going to be OK."

In that moment, I felt as if Dr. Schulz was not just speaking about my medical condition. I felt a deep connection to him and immediately a sense of calmness entered the room. Was this a message that God was sending me? How did Dr. Schulz know for sure that I would be ok? My experience with doctors taking care of my dear mother, for about a decade, never revealed anything more than her doctors expressing optimism, and never the sort of certainty that Dr. Schulz had shown with me.

My faith has always anchored me. My study of the Bible has taught me to ask God specifically for what I want of him. I have learned over the years and have taught that there are benefits to being specific with our requests of God. This has been my belief of a long time. Specific prayers help us clarify our requests. They strengthen our relationship with God and provide the opportunity to bear witness when our prayers are answered.

My unconscious beliefs about cancer collided with my long standing, often spoken, belief that God is bigger than all forms of diseases. Yet, a new and unwelcomed narrative began to unfold in my head. That narrative began to bring on fear, doubt, guilt, sadness, and a massive dose of disappointment. *What was I going to do in this moment of uncertainty and distress?*

Surely, I could not go to God with all of this. What is He going to think of me? What did God expect of me in this moment? Was I going to be led by the human condition alone and not tap into the faith that I had practiced for much of my adult life?

Barbara, this is your most defining moment. This thought began to play on perpetual loop in my mind. I asked myself: *What do you really believe? What do you want?*

At this moment, darkness began to creep in. Self-judgement had free reign over me. I started to relive every bad decision I had ever made in my life; like the decision to take a short cut through a dark but familiar alley at night, to go to the store, as a teenager. This did not turn out well for me at all. Then there was a decision I made to tell a lie that ruined a valued friendship in my early twenties. Every mistake, many of them, began to weigh on me. The self-condemnation became overwhelming.

In the stillness, when my family had given me some space, I knew this was not the time for a superficial talk with God. Like father Abraham appeared to be bargaining with God on behalf of Sodom and Gomorrah, in Genesis 18:16-33, I desired to be emboldened to ask God at least one frank question. In no way did I want to really bargain with God. To bargain with God would mean that I would have to believe that I had something God wanted and could not get without me. That is not my belief. To the contrary, I believe everything belongs to and is controlled by God.

What then was so difficult and why did I feel so far away from God's presence? Finally, I realized that since I received the cancer diagnosis, I had not invited God into my crisis. Jeremiah 33:3 says, "Call to me and I will answer you, and will tell you great and hidden things that you have not known."

I knew that God wanted me to depend on Him and to demonstrate that dependence through prayer and acknowledgement. "And, call upon me in the day of trouble: I will deliver thee, and thou shalt glorify me," Psalm 50:15. It was time to simply open my mouth and my heart to God. It was time to invite Him into the situation. It was time for me to ask God what He thought about the matter of my having breast cancer. He promised to hasten His word unto performance in my life. I had no reason to believe that He would not keep His promise.

I finally could pray this healing prayer sent to me by Gael T. Davis:

The Healing Prayer

God of all creation. You who spoke a simple command and brought forth light from the darkness. I call upon you now to send forth your miracle working power into every aspect of my being, in the same way that you spoke unto the dust of the ground when you created humankind in your own image.

I ask that you send forth your healing power into my body. Send forth your word and command every cell, electrical and chemical impulse, tissue, joint, ligament, organ, gland, muscle, bone and every molecule in my body to come under complete and perfect health, strength, alignment, balance and harmony. It's through you that I live, move and have my being.

With every breath that I take, I live under your life-giving grace and mercy. I ask you to touch me now, with the same miracle working power that you used when you fashioned me inside my mother's womb. And surely, as you have created me in your image and likeness, you can also recreate me now and restore my health.

8 RESTORATION

> *Please fill me with your healing power. Cast out all that should not be inside of me. I ask you to mend all that is broken. Root out every sickness and disease, open all blocked arteries, rebuild my internal organs, rebuild my damaged tissues, remove all inflammation and cleanse me of all infections, viruses and destructive forms of bacteria.*
>
> *Let the warmth of your healing love flood my entire being, so that my body would function the way it was created to be, whole and complete, renewed in perfect health. I ask this through my Lord Jesus Christ, your son, who lives and reigns with you and the Holy Spirit, one God forever and ever.*
>
> AUTHOR UNKNOWN

Everything shifted for me. I could feel the weighted cloud of fear dissipating. That was an answer to my prayers. In an overarching way I knew I was covered, and I felt relief because my prayers were already being answered.

That relief was good enough for me. It carried me through a major relocation from Los Angeles to Rancho Mirage,

California within 10 days following the diagnosis. It allowed me to immediately close my coaching practice of sixteen years without any anxiety. Not being gripped by fear allowed me to release my Washington, DC apartment, which I used as my DC office, without any reservations. I did not want to break my lease; however, I had a record of written complaints on file concerning the massive delayed construction project going on at the apartment site. I shared the news that I had been diagnosed with breast cancer and could not risk the exposure to the dust and debris from the construction with the property management company. They allowed me to break my lease. Kelsey, my beloved daughter who lived in DC, was able to go in and close it out without any problems.

The new felt freedom, the new home, and the new journey I had embarked on seemed like pieces of a ginormous puzzle. I love working on puzzles and putting them together. My strategy for starting a new puzzle is to always begin with identifying the edges. This would take a lot of time, and most often I would not find them all in the beginning, but find them along the way. Unlike the many puzzles I had put together in the past, this new life puzzle was demonstrably different. Identifying all the edges seemed impossible. This was going to require a different and more radical approach.

My answer came to me in the quiet of the morning as I sat and listened to the deafening silence. The answer I received was that I had to begin with one main piece of this puzzle. This journey would start from the center. God had to be in the center of my journey. His presence in the center of my life was the key to my living or dying, literally and spiritually.

That one piece required only me. Once I identified that main piece, I was free to reach out for help. To my surprise the help was endless; even random at times. This was the beginning of a new awareness for me. I was beginning to discern that I could let go of any thoughts of controlling my future, while embracing the idea that I could co-create and design my way forward with God.

The impact of chemotherapy and other prescribed drugs on my physical body was predictable. I would have significant hair loss, or most likely be left bald-headed. When you look at the photo on the back cover of this book, you can see why I enjoyed my hair. At birth, I had a head full of jet-black thick hair that became an identifying feature of mine as a little girl. A few years ago, on my 57th birthday, I decided that my now silver and black natural curls would become my new identifying feature.

In spite of the very nice comments others made about the shape of my head and how "cute" I looked, embracing my bald head was, and continues to be, difficult. When it's freezing cold and I need a scarf or a hat to keep my head warm, I'm reminded that I'm bald. The sharp pain that I'm forced to endure from bumping my head against a wall or surface when I lean back into something is also an annoying reminder that I have no hair protection on my head.

The next physical hurdle was the decision to have a bi-lateral mastectomy. I did not say the words audibly, but my emotions were screaming, *God do you see what is going on here?*

A double mastectomy was considered the best way to prevent the cancer from showing up again. There would be no breast to nest the cancer. Having had two sizable tumors with lymph node involvement put me at a much greater risk of the cancer returning.

Which woman wants to be flat? In my twenties, I contemplated having breast implants because I did not like being a member of the "itty bitty titty" club. After having my children, things got better, and I was satisfied with the slight increase in my breast size. It never crossed my mind that I could be completely without breasts. But here I was facing the reality of choosing between having breasts or having life. The choice was simple and fast for me although I did not speak it to anyone.

The appointment for the mastectomies was made. It would happen following the three months of chemotherapy treatments, with the hope that the tumors would be much smaller and make for a better outcome of the surgery.

I had only seen one person who had a mastectomy and after three surgeries, she was now talking about having another one that would correct a few things that did not go right the previous times. This really made me nervous. Every "what if" ran through my mind. My team was so confident that Dr. Schulz and Stanley had a full conversation about my options for reconstruction surgery immediately following the mastectomies. They were so sure, it seemed, that I would opt to have reconstruction surgery as so many women do, and not be subjected to the drastic body image of having a completely flat chest.

Following the recommendation of my doctors and family, I made an appointment with the second surgeon to discuss breast reconstruction surgery immediately following the mastectomies.

The way it would have worked was that immediately following the mastectomies, the reconstruction surgeon would step in and begin the second procedure while I was still on the table. The consultation went well, and both Stanley and I felt that this surgeon would be a great choice should I decide to go through with it.

The decision was not so easy for me. I vacillated for days, trying to weigh the benefits of the surgery against the risk of being under the knife for a much longer period of time. I studied and read about other women and the complications associated with having the reconstruction surgery. The most significant account for me was the tremendously rough time my best friend Kathlyn had following reconstruction surgeries. It did not go well for her and ultimately the process was stopped.

I thought of Tshombe Buckman, a young woman diagnosed with breast cancer at 35. Surely, if I were 35 years old and having to make this decision, there would have been less hesitation. This was not my story. I turned 59 years old 2 days after my first chemotherapy treatment. My breasts had served me well. At 13 years old, when they began to protrude, they made me feel like a young woman. At 16, when I wore a size 32 A bra, my breasts made me feel completely grown up, and then at 28 years old when I breast fed my daughter for the first time, I knew they had a much greater purpose.

Without much conversation with Stanley and Debra, but after many conversations with God during my morning walks and my quiet time in bed, I was slowly beginning to make the best decision for me. I considered what the doctors, my family, and a few close friends were saying and finally the answer came to me. I knew what I had asked God for. I asked God for my life. I did not ask Him to save my breasts. My life had never been defined by my breasts and this special season in my life won't be defined by my having breasts either.

Restoration: what was that going to look like for me? Was it going to simply mean that I would feel better for a while only to face the same set of circumstances I was facing now? For as long as I could remember, I had heard about miraculous healings from the Bible and had heard about healings of family members from what seemed now to be minor illnesses, such as colds, headaches, and other chronic pain. In my own life, I had attributed my being able to conceive both my children to a miraculous healing of my body, after two surgeries and spending one full year in an infertility program.

This encounter with breast cancer was remarkably different. Restoration—the returning to the original state—is what I felt deeply in my spirit. It was so intriguing for me to sense the difference between being healed and being restored.

Tshombe Buckman, the woman I referenced earlier, who was diagnosed with breast cancer at the age of 35, shared a part of her story with me.

"The night prior to surgery, I was awakened by what felt like some sort of activity happening within my chest. I can only describe it as a knot unraveling in my breast. As the tightness in my chest unraveled, I could feel something leaving my body—a purging occurring by way of urination. All night long, I woke up releasing whatever was not supposed to be there. I was so tired—almost sleepwalking—but there was a pressing urgency that my body had to follow.

During one of the many visits to the restroom, I heard the Holy Spirit say, 'The cancer is leaving your body,' but I was confused. *What cancer? I don't have cancer! I'm not sick. I'm healthy.* Or so I thought, until the tumor was removed and studied for more observation. Like most people, I was on edge awaiting the results.

After all, most people walk through life wanting to avoid pain. It's our natural inclination to stay away from anything that might hurt us. By design our biological make-up has a built-in 'fight or flight' mechanism that helps us navigate through such confrontations."

Hearing Tshombe's story really made me think about how deeply personal God wants to be with us and how His presence in our lives and our affairs is so personal and private. Knowing God's voice and recognizing when He is speaking with us and working on our behalf is essential to both healing and restoring. I was clear about what I heard. I was clear that God wanted to restore me and wanted to use me for something much greater than I could imagine. Surrendering completely to this knowledge was my intention, but it was a new and difficult practice for me.

My fear of an unsuccessful surgery was great. I was afraid I could be left deformed and without the use of my arm. I was not thinking about dying. I was thinking about living as a mutilated woman. In no way was this thought connected to how I felt about my surgeon. Yet, the powerful force of that negative narrative had gotten around my intention to completely trust that God was in control.

At this point, I believed I would survive the cancer. I did not think that I was going to die. My son Cody felt the same way. He shared with me his fear that I would be sick for a long time and would take too much prescribed medicine rather than CBD oil as he recommended. (CBD stands for cannabidiol. It is the second most prevalent of the active ingredients of cannabis marijuana). My concern was about the quality of my life post-surgery. It probably was not helpful that I logged in hours during the middle of the night on YouTube. I looked at hours of videos of other women's experiences, some good, but most not so good. I finally had to stop myself from watching the scary ones that did more harm than inform me. All of this visual information locked inside of my thoughts, along with the friends who had gone through their own experiences, and had shared the details with me, began to impact me greatly. I did not share this with Debra or Stanley, knowing they would have shut that access down immediately.

For most days, Stanley and Debra concentrated on helping me get through the rough chemo experience. The treatments lasted from January 6th through March 28th. It was an aggressive schedule for an aggressive disease that wanted to destroy my body as it unfortunately has done to millions of women and men; and will continue to do so until there is a cure. These two earth angels were present every hour of the day, for six months, pre- and post-surgery. They never left me alone. They took shifts watching over me, serving me, talking to me, and just sitting with me while I cried. My cries out loud were far less than the silent tears that accompanied me as I drifted in and out of sleep most nights. Critical decisions to be made also added to my restless nights.

Effects of the chemo contributed to my not being able to process my thoughts as before, and this was frustrating and at times overwhelming. It was hard for me to confidently state my decision and articulate the reasons why I did not want to have reconstruction surgery. It was so difficult to explain what I was feeling. I thought about how difficult it was to have two C-sections, two years apart, following having one of my fallopian tubes removed to increase my chances of having babies. Three previous major surgeries were seared in my mind forever. Stanley had no way of knowing unless I could tell him that it was too much for me to endure just for breasts.

My babies were the big prizes for going through that unbelievable pain, followed by the horrors of my first baby not coming home for 5 weeks and 13 weeks for my second baby. The prize for going through breast reconstruction surgery would be two artificial bumps, shaped to give the illusion of breasts. Furthermore, there was no guarantee that the surgery would be successful due to the common damage the planned radiation treatment could cause to the implants. I could not wrap my mind around why this would be a good decision for me. I was already on the edge of sanity and constantly seeking ways to keep myself mentally stable.

It was easy to see how some would choose not to go through with all of this and choose something else like checking out altogether. You read the recent statistics about the alarming death rate of women going through this process. This process requires scrappy fight, grit and unshakable faith.

Thank God for lifelines. I had many. The text messages in the middle of the night from my beloved Godmother, Laurie Gibson, seemed to always be right on time. The note cards that came in the mail, (I would open days later) would always have just the right message for the right moment. Sometimes, my lifeline would come in the lyrics of a song on my playlist, as if it was speaking to me in a conversation. One after another, the confirmations of my restoration emerged.

On June 5, 2017, exactly six months from the day I felt the unwelcomed lump in my breast, my oncologist, Dr. Amy Law, said to me during my post operation office visit, "Mrs. Perkins, you are officially a cancer survivor." I hugged her and thanked her. She was so happy for me and my family. She asked about my children and spent more time talking with me about the road ahead as I continued resting and healing from the surgery.

"It is going to take a considerable amount of time to heal. Your body has gone through a lot, but your outcome is much better than many people I see every day. Thank God." A month later I would see my surgeon who would give me the same news!

From that very moment, I understood the responsibility I have to be the living proof that God is still in the restoration business. My testimony would begin with my walk out of the doctor's office. I had the biggest smile on my face and pep in my step. I wanted the patients, new and old, to feel the power of my healing as I walked out. I wanted them to be encouraged by my joy and wanted another woman sitting in that waiting room riddled with fear and uncertainty to grab onto a little hope and keep it with her throughout her journey.

I did have a request for God. I asked for my life, cancer free. He answered YES!

GOD'S PROMISE #1

I will be with you.

"I will instruct you and teach you in the way you should go;
I will counsel you with my loving eye on you."

PSALM 32:8

CHAPTER REFLECTION

Is there something you are asking God to be restored from? What is it?

CHAPTER REFLECTION

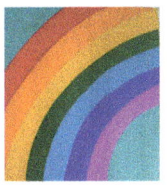

"If you believe, you will receive whatever you ask for in prayer."

MATTHEW 21:22

CHAPTER 2
UNLEASHING THE POWER OF PRAYER

I can vividly remember when prayer was introduced to me as an essential daily part of life. I was seven years old and had moved from Miami, Florida to Nassau, New Providence, Bahamas to live with my Aunt Kathleen. At seven years old, I was too young to understand what moving away from my three other siblings, two first cousins, mother and mother's only sister really meant. Later in life, I came to understand and appreciate that it was such a special gift to my mother for Aunt Kathleen to raise me. It allowed her the freedom to work and care for herself, and the others who were of school age, and much more independent than I was.

Read this excerpt from a sermon by Rev. Beverly Saunders Biddle, a Minister of Spiritual Consciousness and Enlightenment.

Reclaiming Your True Self

"Before we were even formed in our mother's womb, God knew us, and God approved of us. And, when we said "yes" to God's plan, we said "yes" to being God's representative on this earth plane. Somehow, in the process, we lost our way. We forgot why we were called into this existence we call life. We forgot the plan. We forgot our divine connection that can never, ever, be severed. We became enamored with the trappings of this world and placed our faith and trust in human beings, in money, in material possessions, in our image—false as it may be.

It is time for us to return to the place that we only thought we had left. It is time for us to restore our awareness of our connection with our loving, all-providing Creator who formed us in love and who loves us still. It is time for us to reclaim our true selves."

Aunt Kathleen, my great grandaunt, was a praying woman. She had raised my maternal grandfather as her own child, after his mother died in childbirth. When I think about Aunt Kathleen who, at 16 years old, began raising her deceased sister's child and her own child, I could see how prayer became an important part of her life.

My granddaddy used his GI bill to purchase his first home and urged his two daughters to bring their children and come live with him in Liberty City, then a suburb in Miami. It was the American Dream come true for this immigrant who was always a hard-working man. We all lived in a three-bedroom, one bathroom, brick house with three adults and six children. Those were the good old days, where we ate every meal together, prayed together, and played together.

Granddaddy provided childcare for my mother, so I would spend most of my time with him. I was not yet in school, but I was being schooled each day. He was not a religious man; however, he had been raised by Aunt Kathleen. He knew the power of prayer, and at five years old, taught me to say both my grace and my bedtime prayers. They went like this:

Grace
Thank you for the world so sweet,
Thank you for the food we eat.
Thank you for the birds that sing,
Thank you, God, for everything. Amen.

Bedtime Prayer
Now I lay me down to sleep,
I pray the Lord my soul to keep.
If I should die before I wake,
I pray the Lord my soul to take. Amen.

Immediately following granddaddy's funeral service, my mother told me that I was going to be living with Aunt Kathleen in Nassau. She told me that granddaddy loved growing up on that island and living with Aunt Kathleen when he was a boy. That cemented my opinion. I too would be happy like my granddaddy, my best friend, who was now dead. I was not yet sure what that meant. His death was the first death I would experience.

Aunt Kathleen was the first person I knew who genuinely prayed without ceasing. Early on, I thought she was simply old and a bit strange. It took me forty years to realize that my dear Aunt Kathleen was committed to what she believed. She believed that her life belonged to God and therefore she was in constant communication with Him through prayer and conversation. I am not sure if I understood the difference between her prayers and her conversations with God. However, at times she would ask God a question and quickly follow up with a scripture that would seem to answer the question. Those were the times when I felt she was in conversation with God and using His words from the Bible to answer on His behalf. Even her whispers to God were audible and constant. She thanked Him for everything. She turned over everything to Him and she asked Him for help and forgiveness all throughout the day. Living with her for 10 years, I never knew one day when she was not in prayer or conversation with God. I also learned the difference between being in prayer and being in conversation with God.

Aunt Kathleen prayed for others by name when she knew their names and by description when she did not. Sometimes, I would get confused by her calling the names of people she absolutely did not like in her prayers. My young mind wondered why she brought bad people into her good prayers. At seven years old I did not fully understand the power, nor did I really understand the purpose, of prayer. I knew that Aunt Kathleen always believed that God would do as He promised to do. I witnessed what it meant to hang onto God's word and believe Him with all your heart. Aunt Kathleen did exactly that. Throughout my life I have desired to have that strong relationship with God, never doubting Him regardless of what the circumstances may be.

When we are faced with a life crisis or a major situation, our capacity to remember is deepened. We often examine ourselves more deeply and truthfully when in search of solutions. I heard a rather powerful message from a television minister once that said, "The secret to our future is hidden in our daily routine." My daily routine included prayer. However, as I examined this daily practice while seeking healing from cancer, I realized that my prayers were inconsistent and routine. I realized that I had not unleashed the true power of prayer in my life.

I needed fervent prayer in my life. Fervent means to have an elevated level of intensity and enthusiasm. James 5:16 says, "The effectual fervent prayer of a righteous man availed much." James is making the point that intensity and passion is required by the righteous. He teaches that we must do more than simply go through the motions, offering routine prayer that lacks passion.

God sent me exactly what I needed almost immediately after gaining this awareness. The telephone calls began to come in. They were from men and women from around the country, who had heard about my diagnosis from others or from a Facebook post I made the week before my chemotherapy treatments began.

I had a few reasons for posting about my situation on Facebook. I wanted to share news with people I believed cared about my well-being. I wanted those who believed in prayer to pray for me and to do so by name and with a desire to witness my healing. I did not want to buy into the shame of being ill, as if cancer was a punishment for something I did.

When I was growing up in The Bahamas, I rarely heard of anyone having breast cancer. The few times that I remember hearing about anyone having cancer, it was in a whisper and never with details. All I would hear was that "she has cancer." I never heard what type or where it was or that it was something a person could live with or survive. Cancer, to me growing up, was a mystery disease that some poor unlucky person got and would die from because there was no known cure.

When my favorite cousin Pamela found out that I had cancer, she began to pray for me because that is what praying women do. However, she shared with me when she saw me a few weeks after I had been in months of treatment, that she had not seen anyone completely cured. For the most part, what she saw was people dying or only cured for a time, and then the cancer would return. The restoration that I was speaking about, she had not witnessed. However, she prayed for me to be restored anyhow and continues to pray for me.

Many of the calls I received ended with believers asking to pray for me. There were a few calls that came regularly. Gael T., my dear friend for 25 years, wanted to know my treatment schedule so that she could call me on the morning of treatment day. She did. Gael led me in prayer before every chemo session, reciting a healing prayer. I have shared that prayer with others and prayed for the healing of others with this prayer. Dr. Barbara William Skinner, a noted spiritual leader and author of the book, *I Prayed, Now What?* called me monthly and prayed with me. She added my name to a national prayer list, and I began to get calls from individuals associated with that call. Rev. Leah Daughtry, called on a day when I was feeling low in spirit. She talked with me, prayed with me and within days sent me a beautiful prayer shawl that she had crocheted. I would wrap myself in this shawl and pray. This precious gift is still on my writing chair in my prayer room.

My beloved God-sister, Tammilee Jules, had been one of my devoted prayer partners for years. Every telephone conversation was a prayer. Tammilee's greetings were prayers and her goodbyes were prayers. She has a way of infusing God and prayer into every situation and this time was even more intentional. Regardless of how I felt, receiving a call from Tammilee was welcomed. Tammilee knew first-hand about the power of prayer and how prayer is the gateway to our healing. She had been diagnosed with HIV. Most people believed her life would have been over long ago, but it had been 20 years since her first diagnosis. God had healed her, and she believed he would heal me.

The night I found the lump in my breast, I had come home from my first face to face advisory board meeting for the Howard University School of Business, MBA Program. It was a successful dinner meeting. I met some extremely nice people, two of whom I knew I would follow up with immediately. Elliot Johnson, the Chair of the advisory board was one of them. He was interesting, and I sensed he was a man of faith simply by the way he conducted himself at the meeting and his demeanor. I wanted to get to know him better and find out how I could be effective on the board.

The board follow-up did not happen, but early one morning only a few weeks after my diagnosis was made public, I received a call from Mr. Johnson. At first, I did not know who he was, because we had only met that one time at dinner. He had to repeat his name and where he was from to help me remember. Once I remembered, I became a bit emotional when he asked to pray with me. He shared that the Executive Director, Kim Wells, had told him of my medical situation and that he called to encourage me and pray with me. He shared that he had a testimony about how God can heal and wanted me to know about it during my season of health challenges. What a special gift it was to receive these types of calls.

I did not anticipate the overwhelming positive impact that these prayer calls would have on me. Hundreds of people began praying for me daily. My name had been placed on prayer lists and with prayer groups as far as Ghana, Africa. Since we had moved to Rancho Mirage, California, social media apps allowed me to receive calls through my laptop computer.

The unexpected calls frequently brought me to tears. There were some people with whom I reached out to because of their anointing and gift of prayer. One day, I was preparing for a mega regiment of chemotherapy. Chemo sucks! That is the best way to describe it. A cocktail of poison was going to be infused into my body at high doses. Prayer was what I needed. I called Dwan Fortier and her husband Nate. She prayed a most powerful prayer for me. Dwan knew a lot about praying for healing. Her husband Nate had a stroke while celebrating their anniversary over 10 years ago. Prayer pulled him through many emergency hospitals stays and relapses. Prayer brought Nate from not being able to communicate at all to being able to be my friend on Facebook and communicate with the world through social media. Dwan knew something about the type of prayers I needed.

Prayer was my response when people asked if there was something, they could do for me. Bishop Sherman Gordon, Pastor Sandra Crouch, Pastor James Adams, Pastor Zina Pierre, Pastor Thurman Evans, Reverend Shaheerah Stephens, Mama

Iya, Reverend Beverly Biddle, Reverend Lori Billingsley, and Prayer Warriors: Laurie Gibson, Tammilee Jules and Gladys Martin, I thank God for you. This exceptional group were intercessors on my behalf.

I believed from the depth of my being that the collective prayers of this small army of prayer warriors would make a difference in how the chemo would impact my life. Gael T. decided that we would change the name of the concoction to "Jesus Juice." I must admit that I could not hear Jesus associated with anything about this infusion, but later I began to call it that and see it as a positive dose of Jesus Juice being sent in to destroy the bad cells in my body.

Random acts of kindness were starting to become the norm during the early weeks into treatment. At the urging of my son, Cody, I sought out a yoga class nearby. Cody recommended yoga and insisted that it would help me recover from the harsh weekly treatments. I was drawn to the name, "Desert Yoga Therapy," because it suggested healing treatment. After a brief telephone conversation with Jayne Robinson, the owner and primary yoga instructor, I signed up for my first ever Restorative Yoga Class beginning the very next day.

I began attending twice a week and was in love with going to the classes before the treatment began. I shared with Debra, who shared with my best friend from college, Leslie Davis, how much I loved going to yoga and especially how much I appreciated being in Jayne's class. Leslie and a few of my college classmates got together and gifted me months of classes with Jayne. This was so kind. Leslie, Stephen, Kim, Nanci and Marleen gifted me something that is now a part of my life's practice.

It was a Wednesday morning class, I was feeling highly emotional and a bit anxious, thinking about the upcoming chemo treatment in two days. It was also the week that my hair had fallen out completely, as well as my eyebrows. There is no way to prepare for having this happen to you. Looking in the mirror that Wednesday morning was difficult. I did not feel good nor did I look good. The class was small, maybe six others. I had arrived just a few minutes prior to the start time and wanted to head to the back of the room, but the back row was taken. I took the mat in the center of the room, directly in front of the instructor. This added to my anxiety. I truly did not want to be seen, but I wanted the benefits of being in that class and listening to Jayne's calming voice.

We began in a very simple pose, lying on the mat facing up, in what felt like the perfect surrender position. I was comfortable, and Jayne would make sure we were all comfortable. With my eyes closed, I could feel Jayne's energy getting closer as she moved from person to person, asking to help support them in getting even more comfortable. She would routinely go around the room asking if we wanted a blanket or no blanket. This was the best part for me as a new student. I loved being covered up by Jayne with the blanket. She took such good care of us. She would adjust the blanket just right and support our heads and arms with more blankets. I had never experienced anything as comforting as this before.

It was my turn, and Jayne could already see the tears running down my face. I had to remove my eye cover and was pulling Kleenex from inside my blouse, where I had stuffed them just in case I needed them. It was that kind of morning, and I knew it would not take much for me to have an emotional experience. Jayne was extra gentle, and I assured her that I was really okay, just releasing some emotions. She fussed over me in her usual manner, but when she asked that I raise my head a little so that she could provide me a little more support with another blanket under my head, my scarf slipped off, exposing my bald head for the first time in class. I stopped breathing.

I believed the others were fully into their practice, however I became overcome by shame and sadness. The tears were quiet, but uncontrollable. There was nothing that Jayne should have done differently. This was a moment that needed to happen. I was cared for and attended to in every way. It was an answer to a prayer that I could release all of the bottled-up feelings that I tried to hide with my head scarf. I felt exposed, uncovered, yet free. The experience took me so much higher in my consciousness. The wide swings in my emotions from happy to sad, from clarity to complete confusion. Distress was expected in these months of treatment. Having cancer was stressful and some days too much to handle. Cody was right! Yoga was an answered prayer.

I cannot remember all the names of those who prayed for me. Truthfully, I do not know all the hundreds of people who prayed for me. What I do know is that their prayers were answered. Prayers unleashed saved my life. God knew I would need to have a strong foundation, supported by a solid prayer life and belief system. This plan was in place and being implemented from the first day when my beloved Aunt Kathleen showed me how to get on my knees and pray. In the same manner that she prayed about everything, I prayed about every aspect of my treatment, as well as my life beyond the treatment.

I would pray for my doctors and for the medical team working in any way on my behalf. I prayed over the medicine, asking God to take away the side effects and prayed for the instruments that were being used on me that they would be free of germs or harmful bacteria of any kind. I prayed for traveling grace driving to and from the cancer center and prayed for those waiting in the center for their treatment. Silently, prayer became my obsession. It was as if I had become that same old and a bit strange woman of God that I saw in Aunt Kathleen at seven years of age.

Prayer changes things. This is not a cliché. It is a promise to those who believe that God has proven time and time again, that His promises will be fulfilled. Prayer without works is dead. This means that with prayer, there has to be faith in seeing the outcome as God would see it.

Pastor, Lori George Billingsley, a dear friend and woman of God, reminded me of the woman with the blood issue. A story found in the book of Matthew, Chapter 9. This woman was healed after 12 years of suffering. This woman had a strong faith and determination to do something she had not ever done before- touch Jesus. That was "the works" part that accompanies faith. I believe we can touch Jesus through our prayers.

God always answers our prayers, even if we do not like the answer. He never ignores His own. How and when God answers our prayers is also His business. No matter what the situation is, we cannot hasten God. Dr. Barbara William-Skinner says, "We pray not to get what we want from God, but we pray to get God." His view of every situation in our lives is much more expansive. He sees around every curve and far into the future. Prayer makes the future worthwhile in that it is the planting of the seeds of hope and faith.

What in your life requires the kind of prayer I am writing about? Have you really prayed or are you still thinking about it? Do you feel you are worthy of the outcome you are praying for? Is there something standing between you and your prayers to God? What will it take to remove what might be in the way?

Listen my friend, maybe you have prayed like this before and maybe that prayer was answered, but here you are again in need of help. Do you know that God forgives everything and everyone? He is that father who is anxious to forgive us for all things. He simply wants to have a good relationship with us. He waits for us to come to Him as He has taught us in Psalms 23:

> "The LORD is my shepherd; I shall not be in want. He makes me lie down in green pastures, he leads me beside quiet waters, He restores my soul. He guides me in paths of righteousness for His name's sake. Even though I walk through the valley of the shadow of death, I will fear no evil, for you are with me; your rod and your staff, they comfort me. You prepare a table before me in the presence of my enemies. You anoint my head with oil my cup overflows. Surely goodness and love will follow me all the days of my life, and I will dwell in the house of the Lord forever." Amen.

My divine inheritance would not be cut off because of cancer. This was at the root of my prayers. My divine inheritance is ensured in spite of cancer because of the prayers unleashed on my behalf. In my all-day conversations with God, we are not just talking about breast cancer, we are talking about His unlimited blessings in my life and the lives of those around me. My talks with God are prayers. The songs I sing about God are my prayers. The zest I feel in my body when I think of His goodness are my prayers. Unleashing the power of prayer, interjecting God in good times and rough times, and always expecting a miracle are my greatest life lessons. This is what my encounter with breast cancer has done for me. Cancer became a teacher for me. Cancer reminded me that a life without prayer is empty.

This is my prayer for you:

> *Dear God, our Father who knows everything before we open our mouths to speak about our circumstances, thank you for listening. Thank you for being the one we can come to when all else seems useless and often hopeless. I am asking you today to hear my petition on behalf of your beloved child who at this very moment is weakened in spirit and strength. As written in the book of James, we are to confess our sins to each other and pray for each other so that we may be*

healed. My prayer is for restoration in the life of your child. Whatever the situation dear God, you are able to recreate it, change it and turn it around. God, we promise to give you all the glory and praise. In Jesus name. Amen.

GOD'S PROMISE #2

I will give you strength.

"But you, Lord, do not be far from me. You are my strength; come quickly to help me."

PSALM 22:19

CHAPTER REFLECTION

Take some time to write about your situation. What role will prayer have as you confront this challenge in your life? Do you know how to pray? Do you have a prayer partner? How can I support you in your prayer life? Make a call today for help to someone you know who has a strong prayer life.

_____

_____

_____

_____

_____

CHAPTER REFLECTION

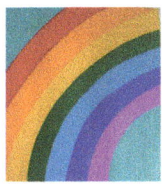

50 RESTORATION

CHAPTER REFLECTION

"Do not conform any longer to the pattern of this world, but be transformed by the renewing of your mind. Then you will be able to test and approve what God's will is— His good, pleasing and perfect will.

ROMANS 12:2

CHAPTER 3
TRANSFORMATION

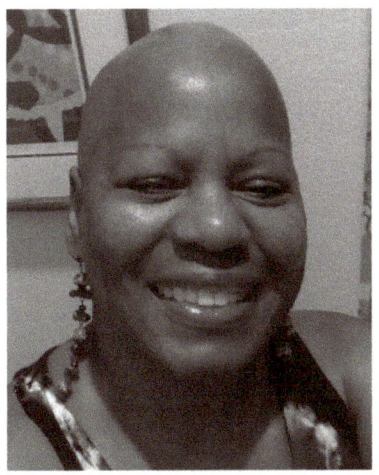

"Change the way you see the thing and the thing
you see will change."

BARBARA A. PERKINS, M.A.

Although I had heard variations of this idea numerous times, it resonated with me like never before. I was about to undergo my last chemotherapy treatment with Dr. Shultz, who was also scheduled to perform my bilateral mastectomy on May 22, 2017.

It was no coincidence that I had been in Bible study with a small group of women whom I referred to as my prayer partners. We began slowly reading the book of Genesis on January 2nd, 2017. Here we were in May, reading the last chapters, covering Jacob's sons who had disappointed him so deeply by hurting their brother Joseph and selling him into slavery. The brothers of Joseph harbored such bad feelings for him that they allowed their father Jacob to believe that his favorite son was dead, perhaps eaten by wild animals. We studied that, in fact, Joseph had been elevated to the highest possible position in the land all the while separated from those he loved. Throughout his many unfortunate ordeals, he remained faithful to God.

When united with his brothers, who themselves believed he was dead, Joseph showed them great compassion and love. He could have held so many things against them. He could have hated them and despised being in their presence. Instead, Joseph did the unimaginable. He loved them, forgave them, honored them and treated them as family. Joseph changed the way he saw his brothers' past bad deeds and immediately those bad deeds were no longer the center of his world.

> *"Change the way you see the thing and the thing you see will change."*

My feelings about cancer paled in comparison to how much I was afraid of actually being diagnosed with it. As I reflected on how much had changed in my life in such a short amount of time, I began to reflect on the behaviors of women I witnessed growing up when one among them was believed to have cancer. The strongest impression about that time was feeling the emotional pain from isolation.

Getting a cancer diagnosis was not a common occurrence when I was growing up. Therefore, when it happened death was presumed certain. Admittedly, this was not what I wanted to believe, but within hours of being diagnosed I could sense the deadly fear that was beginning to occupy a much larger space in my consciousness. *Oh, dear God, not cancer,* I thought, forcing myself to continue breathing.

Then, as if pre-planned, I was the Bible study reader on the day that the text revealed how Joseph had a renewal of his mind about his rogue brothers. He completely shifted the way he felt about his drastic situation. For me this was the tangible example of how I could shift my secretly embedded beliefs about cancer to something completely different.

> "Change the way you see the thing and the
> thing you see will change."

This phrase seemed to now be on a loop in my head. For sure I am going to die. However, I do not have to die from breast cancer.

Before I was diagnosed, thoughts of dying were not a preoccupation of mine. I knew then, and now, that death is inevitable. I had to decide if was I going to allow myself to be dragged around by my emotions or if I was going to be open-eyed about what was at work. Life, and everything associated with it, both the good and the bad, happens. This indeed was no time for me to ignore the emotions that were beginning to surface. This was the time for me to purge negative thoughts from the root to avoid the contamination they would continue to cause in my life. I knew that negative thinking had no history of serving me or anyone else well. This fact was reiterated by Dr. Law, my oncologist. She told me that a major part of getting rid of the cancer from my body depended on my attitude while being treated. I knew I had some transformative work to do and I intended to do it quickly.

There was no shortage of women that I could call on to ask about their battle to overcome a cancer diagnosis.

According to a 2016 article,* from Centers for Disease Control:

"Black women and white women get breast cancer at about the same rate, but black women die from breast cancer at a higher rate than white women."

There are further studies that find the rates of deaths vary from city to city. An article from WebMD, "African American Women: Breast Cancer More Deadly?" October 28th, 2012, states that in a study which looked at breast cancer deaths between 2010 and 2012, in the 43 most populous U.S. cities,

---

* LC Richardson, SJ Henley, JW Miller, G Massetti, CC Thomas, "Pattern and Trends in Age-Specific Black-White Differences in Breast Cancer Incidence and Mortality-United States, 1999-2014," (*MMWR Morb Mortal Wkly Rep* 2016;65:1093-1098), DOI: http://dx.doi.org/10.15585/mmwr.mm6540al.

African American women are 43 percent more likely to die from breast cancer than Caucasian women. The study researcher Marc. S. Hurlbert, PhD, of the Breast Cancer Research Foundation in New York states, "these are shocking and alarming numbers." These numbers are worse than a similar study,[*] conducted in 2009, which showed the difference in death rates was 39.7 percent.

The study went on to show that in 42 of the 43 cities examined, African American women die from breast cancer at higher rates than white women. In Boston, women of both races die at about the same rate. In Atlanta, the findings were "startlingly high." It was noted that African American women are dying of breast cancer at a rate surpassed double that of white women. These findings are according to the Avon Foundation, which funded the study.[**] The top 10 cities with death disparities from breast cancer found in this study are:

---

[*] Kathleen Doheny, "African American Women: Breast Cancer More Deadly?," WebMD, last modified October 28th, 2012, https://www.webmd.com/breast-cancer/news/20121028/breast-cancer-african-american-women#1.

[**] Sinai Urban Health Institute and Breast Cancer Research Foundation Funded by the Avon Foundation for Women, "Black: White Disparities in Breast Cancer Mortality in the 50 Largest Cities in the United States, 2005–2014," accessed on July 1, 2019, https://www.bcrfcure.org/sites/default/files/

1. Atlanta, Georgia
2. Austin, Texas
3. Wichita, Kansas
4. San Antonio, Texas
5. Kansas City, Missouri
6. Dallas, Texas
7. Memphis, Tennessee
8. Los Angeles, California
9. Oklahoma City, Oklahoma
10. Chicago, Illinois

The article ended with the President of the Avon Foundation, Cheryl Heinonen, expressing her desire to see a "call to action" for ending breast cancer for every woman—not just some.

Tia Morris and I met in the early part of 1991 when our daughters were in kindergarten together at Light and Life Christian School. Our friendship grew almost as fast as our daughters, and our families shared a lot of time together when the children were young. I remember Tia's beautiful mother who proudly attended school events that our children participated in. I also remember that she was a woman of faith and on the ministerial staff at First AME Church in Los Angeles, a church I had visited on many occasions.

It was not until after Tia had gone through her cancer treatment and was at the height of rebuilding her public life that I learned of her personal journey with cancer, which did not begin with her, but with her mother. Our families had not been together for years; ever since the children had grown and were living in other states.

Stanley and I moved to Los Angeles from the San Fernando Valley, where we lived for more than 20 years while raising our children. Tia and I reconnected through Facebook. When she came out to visit me, we sat and talked for two hours, catching up on old times. I sat thinking about how amazingly strong this woman was. She looked great and was healthy. I was so inspired by her courage and fight for life as she told me about her battle with breast cancer. When she left my house, I wept. I wept because it just seemed like so much for one person to endure.

Tia shared her story with me about the decade of helping her mom in her struggles with breast cancer and her consistent faith in God to heal her. Her mother died in September 1992.

Tia and her husband, Percy, were married for ten years. She had advanced in her law enforcement career and was still raising two elementary school aged girls. She had grown concerned about her own health. There was a family history that caused her to begin getting mammograms at 26 years old. That history repeated itself eventually.

In 2006, Tia was diagnosed with breast cancer. She fought like a warrior and continues to fight not just for herself and family, but she is a sought-after speaker on the survivor's circuit. She authored a 364-page testimony of how God is working through her to help others. *Mama's Curse* is Tia's Memoir that tells the story of struggle and survival. Tia was, and still is, one of the women I knew I could call on and I did. She was such a positive voice in the midst of a season that would steal every ounce of joy if you would allow it to.

About 10 days after Stanley and I had packed up and moved from Los Angeles to Rancho Mirage, California, a beautiful suburb just east of Palm Springs, I sent Tia a direct message via Facebook. It included my diagnosis. I shared that we had moved about 5 miles from the Eisenhower Lucy Curci Cancer Center, in Rancho Mirage, where both my oncologist and surgeon worked. I asked her to give me a call because I wanted her help and had a few questions that I knew she would be able to answer. Tia's response was quick, compassionate, and full of concern for my well-being. She immediately offered to come to Palm Springs to help me. She offered a prayer in her voice mail and promised to reach out again soon. She did and was so helpful to me all along the way. I felt the need to be connected to women who knew the terrain I would be confronted with. I wanted to be able to call for help from women who knew what I would need before I asked.

There were days over the course of three months and eight rounds of chemo where I thought the treatment was just too much to bear. The drugs were awful. Neulasta®, in particular, had its way with me. The pain was debilitating and seemed to suck the life from my body. Everything I did required more physical strength than I had. Talking, walking, brushing my teeth, and using the bathroom were all so exhausting. Taking a shower was so strenuous that I would have to immediately go straight to bed.

The ladies, Tia, Kathy, and Julia warned me about fatigue. I had actually witnessed an episode of fatigue with Kathy when she was going through her treatment a few years prior. We had gone out to a formal dinner in Washington, DC, where President

Obama and First Lady Michelle were the keynote speakers. Armando, Kathy's husband, warned us that it might be too much for her. We planned the outing so carefully with every detail in place. Kathy's hotel room was within walking distance from our seats. We arrived early the day before the event in order for her to be well rested. We avoided the temptation of shopping with our favorite vendors so that we could preserve Kathy's strength for the dinner. This was going to be our night out just like old times. We paid attention to all the details, like having the air conditioner as low as possible while getting dressed and of course, factored in breaks. We were not going to take any chances with her overheating.

We made it to the dinner and were so proud of ourselves. Kathy looked stunning. We were having such a good time the hour before the dinner started. We were there early because we did not want to be rushed in the middle of the crowd while going through the security check-in process. Being early made for a longer evening and more hours that Kathy would be up and moving.

Then it happened. The energy and excitement at the table was high. We were all snapping pictures, taking selfies and waiting for a sign that the Obamas were in the building. I did not take my eyes off of Kathy for too long. She was doing fine, and we all were as happy as ever. We were having fun, just like old times, before her diagnosis.

Then, I noticed that Kathy's smile was suddenly gone, and she was not talking. I quietly asked her how she was doing. Her response was with a nod and a half smile. I knew something was happening but was not prepared for how quickly the situation would change. She asked me to help her get to the ladies' room and I did. Before we could get there, I could see the physical change that was happening. Her face was drenched with perspiration; she was labored as she tried to walk in her heels. Her walk was not steady, as she noticeably wobbled from side to side. Many thoughts raced through my head. What was I going to do if she fainted?

We got to the restroom so that she could sit, while I called her nephew, the driver, who would show up within minutes. We had planned for this. Fatigue had taken over Kathy's body with little notice. It just happened. This was the fatigue the ladies were now warning me about.

Being with this special group of survivors is my blessing. It did not feel like a blessing early on, however today, I would say it is one of the greatest blessings of my life.

Transformation: *a dramatic change in form or appearance.*

There is no doubt my life and physical appearance have dramatically changed since I defeated breast cancer, but more importantly, I have had an internal transformation. My internal shift has been far more significant and meaningful than what I look like on the outside.

Each day is new. I am intensely aware of my breath. When I wake in the early hours of the morning, I listen for my breath and for my heartbeat. I know that each new day is a gift from God. I know there is a purpose for my being here and that the purpose is in alignment with God's master plan. Cancer came to teach me new things about myself. Cancer came and caused my relationship with God to be deepened. Cancer came and I have been transformed. I see life differently. Everything matters, including the blank spaces in my life. I used to enjoy mindless television watching. Now, I use that time for sending notes to friends and family who might need a word of encouragement. I love Facebook because it allows me to post something uplifting at least once a day with the hope that someone would be helped by what I say.

Cancer came and has prompted me to make enormous shifts in my life. Slowly but surely, I am cleaning up some of the many messes I made along the way. I am seeing broken relationships differently. Now I can see how breakdowns in communication are opportunities for breakthroughs. There is nothing too hard for God. He only asks that we come to Him and lean not on our own understanding of things.

As for the physical changes, I continue to work through the challenges presented each day.

> ***Restoration:*** *The action of returning something to a former condition.*

Being restored meant that I would surrender to being torn down and remade. The tearing down part is painful. I began writing this chapter with the statement that I have to repeat to myself, as a way to encourage myself from time to time. I am Barbara Perkins. I am bald, breastless, and beautiful.

This statement has helped me on many occasions while getting dressed in the privacy of my bathroom. Dressing for special events does not have the same feeling it did before cancer. I

An access port placed and implanted for treatments and to take blood.

MEMORIES

My nails turned black, a side effect of chemotherapy.

love fashion. I love getting dressed up for special occasions such as awards shows, formal dinners, and parties.

I read an article some time ago that said, "body image is a person's perception of the aesthetics or sexual attractiveness of their own body." This was not the first time in my life when I struggled to appreciate how I looked. Growing up, I had a gap between my two front teeth. I did not like it and never felt that it was attractive. I was forty years old when I finally got braces to close it. There are times now when I look at old photos of myself that I actually miss having that gap. My hair also presented acceptance challenges for me throughout my life. In middle school and high school, I had a head full of thick unruly hair. I endured many days of teasing about my hair. My Aunt Kathleen did not believe in chemical relaxers. We both struggled to keep my hair under control. Aunt Kathleen did not believe in hair coloring either. Therefore, on my 50th birthday, I announced to my husband that I would discontinue dying my hair every two weeks to cover the gray hair that was beginning to overtake the black. At different times in my life, it has truly been a struggle for me to appreciate my look.

Chemotherapy treatments left me bald. My eyebrows and lashes fell off. The bilateral mastectomy (meaning the removal of all the breast tissue from my chest) has left me completely flat chested with two extensive scars that extend from underneath both my arm pits to the center of my chest. Dr. Schulz, my surgeon, did a beautiful job given what was required. Once he was inside, he discovered additional precancerous cells that had to be removed. I could not be more pleased with the outcome of the surgery and the care I was given.

It was solely my decision not to have reconstruction surgery at the same time as the mastectomies. I acknowledge that I do not always feel good about how different my body looks. Those moments are few and pass rather quickly as I encourage myself through gratitude and acceptance. Iyanla Vanzant's message to me and the full audience who attended A Night of Inspiration at Carnegie Hall, was to release the physicality. Stop holding onto what was in the physical and learn to see all things through your spiritual lens.

I am not my hair. I am not my breast. I am the full perfect creation of a masterful God who adores me and has shaped me in His image and likeness.

A dear friend said to me one day when I was having a down moment, "when I am talking with you, I don't think about your

70 RESTORATION

Initial hair loss after starting chemotherapy.

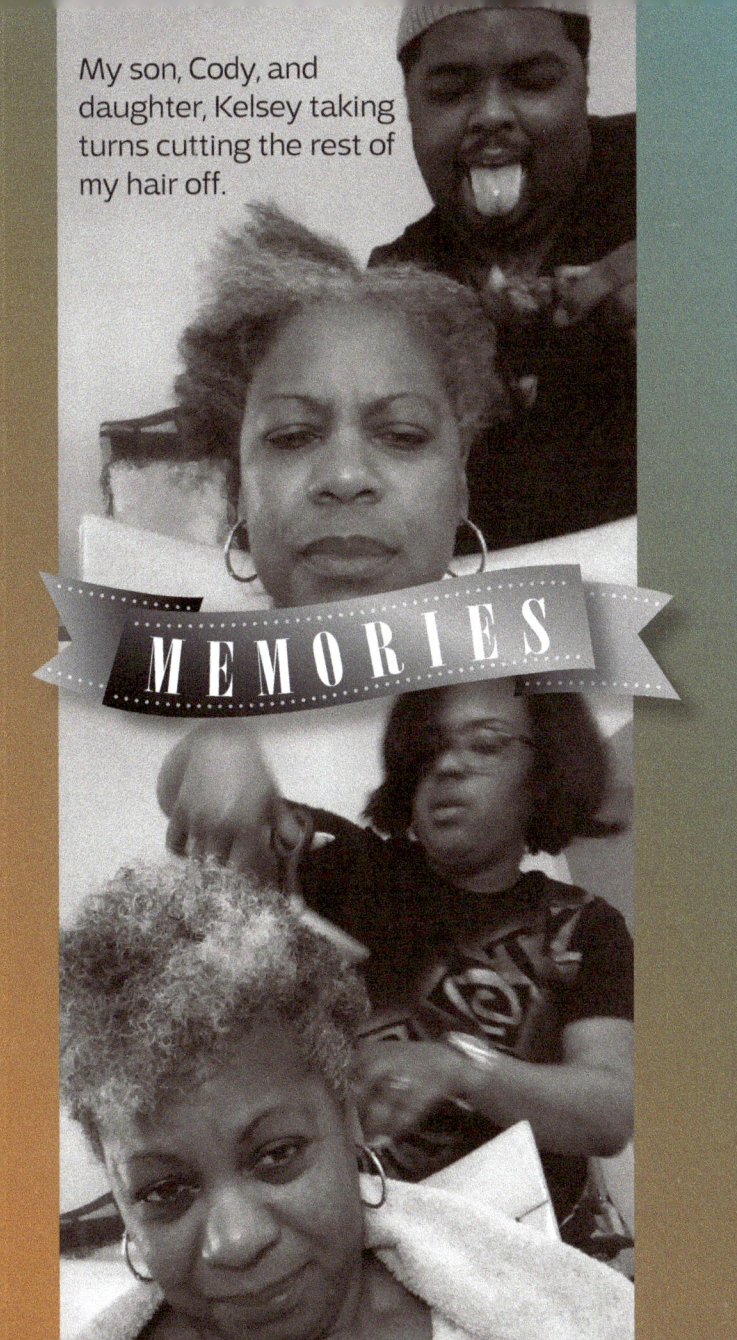

My son, Cody, and daughter, Kelsey taking turns cutting the rest of my hair off.

MEMORIES

hair or the fact that you have no breasts. I am simply happy that we can have a conversation. I am happy you are here."

My response was, "and so am I."

The shifting of my thoughts was the most difficult. How does one remain positive in the midst of suffering? I wanted to believe that there was no way that God would have me suffer. I was beginning to feel like I was suffering. Making the distinction between the pain I was really feeling and the suffering I felt was very important. In reading and researching I found the answer that lead to my mind shift. Deepak Chopra* shared that pain and suffering are not the same:

> "Pain and suffering are not the same." He says, "Left to itself, the body discharges pain spontaneously letting go of it the moment that the underlying cause is healed. Suffering is pain that we hold on to. It comes from the mind's mysterious instinct to believe that pain is good, or that it cannot be escaped or that the person deserves it. If none of these were present, suffering would not exist."

---

* Deepak Chopra, *The Book of Secrets: Unlocking the Hidden Dimensions of Your Life* (New York: Random House, 2004).

Ah ha, this was it for me. Suffering came as a result of my deeply buried belief that I deserved it. I was holding onto the pain for dear life. The more I held onto the pain, the greater the suffering became. The greater the suffering the more pain I felt. How was I going to get off of this roller coaster? I had to get to the root cause of why I believed there was no way to escape the suffering. God was not punishing me. I was punishing me. The question was, why was I punishing me? What had I done that I would choose suffering as the consequence for my behavior?

I wondered if other women felt the way I was feeling. The physical pain was real, and women shared that with me, but no one talked about their relationship with cancer. I did not have the courage to ask them the questions that were coming up from the most secret parts of myself. How was I going to know? I thought about Joseph, from Genesis 37, of the Bible. I thought about the isolation he must have felt during his separation from his family. He must have had the same endless list of questions to which the answers might have been worse than the situation he was in. I acknowledged to myself that some answers would be more painful than the disease. What I needed was to be transformed from the way that I was thinking.

This transformation would be the only way that I could be restored completely. It simply was not possible for me to hold onto the belief that somehow, somewhere, my actions displeased God so much that the only atonement would be my long suffering. I was guilty as charged by myself. How long would I hold onto the guilt? It would take being diagnosed with breast cancer for me to examine what beliefs I was holding onto for years. When I really began to look at snap shots of my life there were infractions upon infractions that I had heaped onto myself, lying dormant in my own personal jail house for troubled souls. *Oh no,* I thought, *this must change. This will change. This is not what God had in mind for me when He created me.*

> "Be renewed by the transforming of my mind? Great, how do I do that? I began to comb my mind for the many lessons I heard as a lifelong student of the Holy Bible. Which lessons would apply to this situation?"
>
> REV. BEVERLY SAUNDERS BIDDLE

Another lesson is found in the story of the penitent thief who would hang on the cross next to Jesus, as written in Luke 23:39-43. The penitent criminal, one of two that hung as Jesus did in pain and suffering, was changed by his experience of being a witness to Jesus's experience on the cross. Unlike the other thief who chose to blaspheme and made fun of Jesus, the penitent thief defended Jesus, proclaiming that he believed in his innocence. He believed that Jesus had the power to save him from the ultimate destruction, so he asked, "Lord, remember me when you come into your kingdom." Jesus accepts his prayer and promises him that he would be with Him in paradise.

In this story, I believe that the penitent thief was transformed with the help of Jesus simply by asking Jesus for help. These were important steps in his process of transformation. The next step would be to believe that transformation was possible even for me.

What do you believe about yourself? What is happening in your life that you need to be transformed from? Does God have the authority in your life to make transformation possible? Do you believe he has the power to do so?

GOD'S PROMISE #3

I will always love you.

"How precious to me are your thoughts, God.
How vast is the sum of them!"

Psalm 139:17

CHAPTER REFLECTION

CHAPTER REFLECTION

"Be kind and compassionate to one another, forgiving each other, just as in Christ God forgave you."

EPHESIANS 4:32

CHAPTER 4
FORGIVE AND FORGET

Growing up surrounded by strong women of faith, I memorized the words of my Aunt Kathleen, "I will forgive, but I am never going to forget." This would apply to whatever the infraction was at the time. Similar versions of this statement I would hear repeated throughout my early years of growing up. They eventually became words that I would repeat as my truth. After all, Aunt Kathleen said them first and she was my first teacher who knew all things. I learned to believe what she believed.

Somewhere in my mid-forties I really began to seek a deeper meaning of truth in my life. I wanted to find the peace that started on the inside and showed up on the faces of those who possessed it. The concept of forgiveness began to open up my curiosity and led me to a series of questions about myself. Had

I forgiven others in my life for things that I believed were their fault? Did I even want to forgive everyone for everything as my spiritual coach and friend Iyanla had suggested? What was I going to do about my loyalty to Aunt Kathleen's beliefs?

When I began to search for my own truth about the subject of forgiveness, I did not have one. What I believed was what Aunt Kathleen believed. If Aunt Kathleen believed as she did, that was good enough for me. Forgiving as Christ forgave us does not mean that we hold onto the memory of the infraction like a battle scar to remind us that the person has the potential to hurt us again. This type of forgiveness is subjective. It is hinged upon a set of parameters that we construct as a benchmark that others must live up to. When they do not, the forgiveness is retracted. The deeper question for me was, how do I forgive those things that seemed impossible for me to forget?

There are a number of hurts in my life that are not ever going to be forgotten, no matter how hard I try. To forget that my innocence was stolen from me as a teenager by someone who betrayed me is never going to be forgotten. To forget that a younger brother, who I raised like my own child, deliberately tried to hurt me and my family, is not something that I can forget. The deep betrayal by a trusted sister-friend that left my character in question will forever reside in that painful memory category. Can I honestly say that I have forgiven in these three examples, where the pain was so great that it felt like physical track marks on my heart? Yes, I have. In my case, time and hours of prayers allowed those old wounds to heal and I could forgive.

I understood how necessary forgiveness was to my own healing. I understood that the residual effects of an unwillingness to forgive spirit could be an unattractive character. This is not what I wanted for myself. I recognized that there are some who look at my life for cues to Christian living and it is extremely important for me to live a life that would not be an embarrassment to God. My character reflects what I believe. An ugly spirit is not how I want others to receive me.

This construct of forgive and forget; I have not found in the Bible. Matthew 6:14 and Ephesians 4:32 teach that we are to forgive others as God has forgiven us. Also, in the book of Matthew we learn that we should forgive those who have sinned against us many times. If we are unwilling to forgive, it has the potential to hinder another's fellowship with God.

Holding grudges against others while seeking to get revenge is not Christ-like. Forgiving others is not optional for living a life pleasing to God. There is no justification for not forgiving others. It is a clear request from God.

Is this difficult? It is arguably the most difficult request that is asked of us as Christians. God asks that we release feelings from the equation and to be obedient without question. When we feel we have been wronged in some way, especially if that wrong falls in the "deal breaker" category, we want to hold on to that wrong. Sometimes, we even get addicted to the pain. If not addicted, we can get stuck in the story as we make a habit of telling it over and over again. The misperception is that if we tell it enough, stay angry enough, we would be able to use that as a shield of protection. The truth is by holding on to hurt we keep it fresh, unintentionally preventing the healing we desire from happening. In fact, we potentially draw that same pain to ourselves again. What we think about we manifest. In the book of Matthew 6:9-10, a believer's mindset is taught. "This, then, is how you should pray:

"Our Father in heaven. Hallowed be your name, your kingdom come, your will be done, on earth as it is in heaven." In Philippians 4:6, "Do not be anxious about anything, but in every situation, by prayer and petition, with thanksgiving, present your requests to God." We learn from Paul, the author, about the benefits of having a God centered mindset.

It is a blessing to be in a marriage for 34 years. It is a special blessing to have been in a relationship with lasting agreements that we are not afraid to modify as time passes. From the beginning of our marriage, Stanley and I made a few steadfast agreements. Perhaps previous relationships taught us that we had to have a plan in place in the event of a marital storm. We both knew that marital storms were likely. Between the two of us, we only saw a few long-term marriages in our families. We were both raised in families headed by strong women who, for the most part, raised their children without consistent help from their husbands. What was the plan for how we would ride out the storms in our marriage?

Stanley's father died just a few years before we met. He represented a norm that was common in the forties. He had two families. In each of these families there were children: three boys with Stanley's mom, his first wife; and four girls with his second wife. There was a period when the three boys, in elementary to middle school, were packed up and sent to live with their father and his second wife. Needless to say, there was some healing and forgiving that had to take place in this situation.

My father, Zebbie Lee Parrish, was nicknamed, "The Duke." The rumor was that the Duke had many "Duchesses." My papa could indeed be characterized as a "rolling stone." Our mothers were hurt in these relationships, yet they seemingly made decisions that benefitted their children. Indeed, there were many benefits to the strength demonstrated by our mothers. However, the overarching lesson was that they forgave the men in their lives and we benefitted in a way that they could not articulate.

Almost 10 years into our marriage my mother came to live with us. She helped us by taking care of our two children while we worked. It was the time when my relationship with my mother grew and I would come to understand some of her life choices better. I saw her, not as my mother, but as a woman who made a strong effort to live a life of peace, provided for her children and trusted in God. My parents, although separated for many years, always remained close friends. One day, my father proudly stated to me that my mother was the only woman he trusted completely. My immediate thought, which I did not have the courage to ask, was: *Why did he hurt her so often?* What I heard in my father's confession to me about my mother was that she was trusted, but perhaps not loved in the way I imagined she needed to be loved by him.

One evening over a glass of wine, sitting by the pool in our backyard, I asked, "Mother, how did you put up with Daddy's cheating?" Her answer surprised me, "He cheated on himself, not me." The response stopped me from asking any follow-up questions. I concluded at the time that Mother was still in denial and maybe even still hurt.

Nothing could have been further from the truth. In hindsight, this is what allowed her to forgive him. Someone who would hurt himself in this way deserved a compassionate heart. Daddy deserved to be forgiven.

However, some years later as they both became more dependent on us, I expressed to Debra, my sister, that since she was caring for our daddy and I was caring for our mother, maybe the two of them could live together. It seemed like a great idea to me, particularly since they were such good friends. Debra allowed me to share that idea with our mother, who once again reduced our conversation to one sentence. "Duke will always be your daddy, but he could never be my husband again." Daddy was forgiven. Mother, while not angry or hurt any longer, had not forgotten the life she lived with our father. That was not a life she wanted to repeat in this stage of her life.

This brings me back to the important question I raised earlier, how do we forgive what seems impossible to forget? Momma Thelma, Stanley's mother and Mother Barbara, my mother, gave tangible examples of how to do this.

The Bible also gives us a very good example in the person of Joseph, found in Genesis, Chapter 37. Joseph was the favorite son of Israel, who wore his famous robe given to him by his father. His dreams of becoming greater than his brothers stirred up extreme jealousy and caused his brothers to sell him into slavery. He was sold multiple times, deeper and deeper into slavery. Over the years Joseph was presumed dead by his family. However, his favor with God allowed his gift as an interpreter of dreams to propel him to become the chief administrator of Egypt.

Later Joseph reunites with his brothers who had betrayed him. Their betrayal hurt him deeply. When the right time came, Joseph reveals that he is their brother and urges them not to be afraid or to feel guilty for betraying him. The reason given to them by Joseph was that the betrayal was all a part of God's plan for his life. God had restored him and given him his family back. Joseph did not forget what his brothers did to him. He forgave them and started a new relationship with them, by first showing his compassionate heart towards them.

It is possible to forgive even those serious violations that we may not ever forget. The Bible states that we should emulate Christ. Ephesians 5:1 says, "Therefore, be imitators of God, as beloved Children." First Peter 2:21 states, "for to this you have been called, because Christ also suffered for you, leaving you an example, so that you might follow in His steps." Luke 6:40 reads, "a student is not above his teacher, but everyone when he is fully trained will be like his teacher."

It is about our daily practice. We can actively pursue forgiveness, but what do we do after we have forgiven?

I will start with what we must not do after we have forgiven. We should not take on the role of detective, working to get to the bottom of the situation. We should not spend time trying to find out what was going on in the head or heart of the violator. What would be the purpose of that exercise? The gathering of facts could only serve to open the wound wider and delay the healing process. Once we have forgiven someone for a hurt, we should not begin to keep a record of past hurts that we will be tempted to pull out if there is ever a need to remind ourselves and others of the past hurts. A book of past hurts will hurt any attempt to recover or reconcile.

If you search for pain, you will find it. As my mother said, cheaters hurt themselves first. Guilt is punishment to me. A guilty mind is a tormented mind. A guilty heart is a tormented heart. I have seen women and men launch a full search and recovery of the worse hurtful evidence you can imagine. In today's society where cameras can be embedded in pens, watches, jewelry, clothing and many other unsuspecting things, it is easy to be seduced by the possibility of having too much information. How do you know when you have gathered enough pain? I asked a client this question once. What do you do with all that hurt that is being gathered? I suspect much of this type of hurt gets buried in our souls and begins to eat away at us from the inside, just like cancer cells. Who would, in their right mind, invite this into themselves? When we are in pain is when we are most aware that we need healing. It is at that moment when our healing practice needs to be engaged.

One of the two agreements I made with Stanley before we were married is that I was not going to police his behavior, nor did I want to be policed. We agreed that if either one of us changed our minds about wanting to be with each other, we would say so. We agreed that respect and protecting each other were high priorities in our marriage. We discussed what the deal breakers would be in our marriage before we were married. This was the best uncomfortable conversation we ever had. What was so good about it was that we only had to have it one time. Over the years, with a few reminders, we certainly have had our trials and challenges, but the two deal breakers, well, thank God we have not had to face. I have forgiven Stanley for many things in 34 years and he has forgiven me perhaps for more.

After forgiveness, if it is possible, aim for reconciliation. There are somethings that would prevent reconciliation and if that is the case forgive and allow God to help you heal your heart.

> "Forgiveness can be granted; restoration can be denied."
>
> Rev. Dr. Howard-John Wesley
> Alfred Street Baptist Church

Don't spend time watching out for repeat offenders. It is not our job to heal them. That's God's job, and His way is always better. Our job is to strive to live above the infraction. Our walk with Christ is higher than any breach of trust, insult, misunderstanding or character assassination.

If you agree that there is some dormant hurt in your life and you feel you are ready to take action to excavate that hurt, I am willing to stand with you. Let me offer this prayer on your behalf first, and then you take it from there.

> *Dear God, who is almighty yet loving and gentle, I am here with your child who has been weighted down with the pain caused by another. God, you know the details of this situation better than we both do. You know why it had to occur dear God. We accept that your way has never been wrong and that somehow good has come in spite of the pain. Thank you, dear Lord, for pointing that out to us. Forgive*

us for holding onto past hurts. Forgive us for not releasing it to you to resolve and taking it into our own hands. God, we trust you with our lives. We believe that you only want what is best for us, so we ask that you remove this burden of anger, hurt, guilt or shame. Take away the sting from this situation dear Lord. Guide me through what feels like an unbearable storm. We believe this prayer is being answered right now. In the name of Jesus, Amen.

GOD'S PROMISE #4

I will give you peace.

"Be still and know that I am God; I will be exalted among the nations; I will be exalted in the earth."

Psalm 46:10

CHAPTER REFLECTION

Take the time to write about what you have released. How will you move forward? What do you need to help you? Now, write about how you feel at this very moment.

_____

_____

_____

_____

_____

_____

CHAPTER REFLECTION

"Before I formed you in the womb, I knew you, before you were born, I set you apart. I appointed you as a prophet to the nations."

JEREMIAH 1:5

CHAPTER 5
DIVINE ASSIGNMENT

It is not by accident that I am writing this chapter while looking out from the balcony of such a beautiful home on Staniel Cay, Exuma, one of the family of islands, in The Bahamas. Nature's music, at 6:30 am, is in the background, penetrating the stillness. I feel like an intruder watching the birds and other exotic creatures gather themselves. They greet each other, as well as the new day. The sun is beginning to light up the sky and I am finding it difficult to speak the words of gratitude that have filled my heart. Many thoughts are racing through my mind in color, one snapshot of God's goodness after another.

There is no question in my mind that grace and mercy have landed me here. I could remember back 50 years ago, while growing up in Nassau, the vision of my going far away to learn and prepare for whatever God had purposed for my life. I intuitively knew that I would be back here, one day, on the land where my ancestors toiled and lived for decades. Waking up in Exuma, on this morning, brought me full circle. My beloved Aunt Kathleen's spirit is very present as I am thinking about the many stories she told me about being a girl child on Staniel Cay.

I am writing this in 2017 and Aunt Kathleen was born in 1910. How do I even imagine what life was like over 100 years ago on this beautiful island? It is beyond difficult to imagine that she sat as I am sitting and thought of me, and my future. She worked toward an invisible dream. Nothing that she did was for her own satisfaction. The well-being of future generations motivated her and the other young men and women of her time. Their footsteps became my life's road map. For this I will be forever grateful.

I am on this beautiful island to celebrate Kathlyn's (Kat) birthday. Kat and Armando's life together has been full of adventure. We all met in 2006, while traveling aboard a cruise ship set to sail the Mediterranean. We have been enjoying life together ever since. The celebration of Kat's birthday grew bigger over the years and became a marker in our lives; especially the last eight years, following her bout with breast cancer. On her 50th birthday I told my sister-friend that God sometimes allows situations to happen to give us a chance to turn to Him and to trust Him deeper than ever before. Now, we both have had the same experience and we have grown closer to each other, and to our God.

Our annual coming together for the birthday celebration is truly a life celebration; a time to give thanks to God for all the good that has happened in our lives. We give thanks to God for all the challenging lessons in our lives and we give thanks to God for giving us the assignment to be the tangible demonstration of His favor. It is not by accident, but by divine appointment that we are together sitting on a veranda that wraps around a beautifully painted island green house, nestled in the hillside of this oasis.

What does God want me to do next? This question has been on a loop in my head since we landed on Exuma. Whatever the assignment is for my life, I am willing to carry it out. Being in the stillness and calm allows me to hear from God in such a sweet way. It also allows me to speak with God in my first voice, the authentic voice that He loves to hear.

Through prayer and meditation, I understand that the assignment for me is multi-faceted. There is an intention for me that is expansive. I believe that God could not have revealed this to me before now. Every experience I have had has led me to this starting point. Thank you God for being such a kind and considerate father. You are such a faithful master teacher in my life. Who, if not God, could have known that there was a shared story that Kat and I would tell? Neither one of us knew that we would be witnesses to the miracle of healing and restoration from such a scary diagnosis.

When I joined Kat's family and friends eight years ago in prayer for her survival, there was not a thought in my mind about having cancer. We prayed for two years as she battled with the emotional and physical harshness of the treatment regimen. Kat shared with me that she had to overcome the fear of death by cancer, burning by fire, or drowning. She had those fears for a very long time. It was not until she allowed her mind to change from cancer being a reason to die, but rather a reason to live. That revelation came as a result of prayer. It was nothing that medicine was able to solve.

My dear friend won her battle with cancer and has been cancer-free for over eight years. The same way I stood with her; she now stands with me. She prays for me and is a confidant I can always depend on. Kat and Armando have been earth angels to my family along this road, helping us to navigate the unknown. I know this is not the end of our story. There are more hills to climb as survivors. We both have become encouragers to other women facing this brutal reality. We both wear our survivor badges as a symbol of victory. This is our divine assignment.

In the past I celebrated, like many others, those special life occurrences such as birthdays, anniversaries, and certain holidays. Now, each and every morning when I realize that God has granted me another day on this beautiful earth, I celebrate with a praise of gratitude. I am thankful for a life of abundance and joy. This divine assignment was created just for me. It was given to me only. God granted me favor and has prepared me to teach and learn simultaneously. The gifts of the spirit are bountiful. The gifts are essential to the work God has for me to do. The only credential I must have to fulfill my divine assignment is a G.O.D. This means God's Official Designation.

Once I became clear about how God works, all worries about what others were doing dissipated. Constantly, I felt God was trying to tell me something. What I needed to know was that I was enough. Everything that I needed for the pathway forward, God had to remind me that I had. The past worry I had about not completing the PhD program I started in 2003 began to be replaced by the knowing that my G.O.D. superseded all other credentialing. The integration of knowledge and wisdom is my newest desire. I pray for the discipline necessary to acquire knowledge that helps to build my confidence. I pray for an endless supply of wisdom to help me navigate the bumps that are sure to come.

> "Service is the rent we pay for occupying our space on the earth."
>
> Anonymous

This is such a powerful statement to live by. Another moving statement that I have tried to remember as I walk through life is, "the dash between your arrival date on the earth and your departure is what defines you." What are the stories that others would tell about you once you have made your transition? What did you co-create with God? What works have you done to help improve the lives of others?

The creator of the universe has already done the most difficult parts. It was God alone who flung those bright, beautiful stars in the skies over Exuma. It was God alone who created the oceans that separate us on one side and brings us back together on the other. It was God who dreamt this perfect world, allowing us to participate as we do daily. He watches how we participate in our own restoration. He seasons our hearts through these life situations. He listens for our whispers back to Him affirming our desire to be His earthly hands and feet.

Two months post-surgery, I attended weekly physical therapy sessions to help me regain better use of my right arm. The muscles were cut deeply during my surgery, and the removal of the lymph nodes resulted in a weakened arm. An important lesson that came from this experience was to allow others to help me. My faith in the entire human experience increased once I was in acceptance of others and allowed them to share in this experience with me. The small and petty differences became smaller as the small acts of kindness became bigger in my life.

No area of my life was overlooked. Every part of me was put to the test. The forgotten mishaps and brushes with family members resurfaced seeking to be healed. Nothing could stand in the way of my pleasing God, therefore, everything had to be surrendered. Freely, I wanted to address any and all things that would threaten my relationship with God. Nothing could stand in the way of my carrying out my divine assignment. The old habits that ceased to serve me for my highest good had to change. I am as ready now as ever before to live my best life.

I have faith as a companion through rough times. Faith reminds me that I was chosen by God to be His servant, in service for Him. Faith is stored for the times when it is most needed. God cares more about the intentions of my heart than the mistakes of my hands. The emphasis in my life is on the victories, not the failures. I don't look like my challenges. I look like my victories because I have faith. Every day God provides a road map for me to follow through the studying of His word.

> "Therefore, with minds that are alert and fully sober, set your hope on the grace to be brought to you when Jesus Christ is revealed at His coming. As obedient

children, do not conform to the evil desires you had when you lived in ignorance. But just as He who called you is holy, so be holy in all you do; For it is written: "be holy because I am holy."

1 PETER 1:13-16

I believe everything about my life is by design. I believe the same about you. There is a purpose for your being here. Our lives are not accidental. How we get to our purpose is a solo experience that will unfold when we let God know that we are ready to hear Him. Life is such a special gift we have each received. Let us show our utmost gratitude for this gift. Let us show that we know how different it could have been if not for the love, grace and mercy of God. I want to be the receiver who shows unmatched gratitude for the most special gift in the world, which is to receive the love of God that He so freely gives to me.

Cancer had the potential to steer me away from what God intended for me to do with the rest of my life, but I fought cancer like a girl and picked up the broken pieces as an offering to God Almighty. Now this new road is full of such excitement each day. My assignment is to be a witness to the unimaginable power of God. My territory has been enlarged and I have been blessed beyond what I have asked for. Writing this book and being able to share this testimony with thousands, is part of the assignment He has for me. The success of this book will lead to the increase that He promised if I would obey Him by seeking Him first above all else.

You have an assignment my friend. Do you know what it is? What are you willing to co-create with God? Do you have a spiritual daily practice? Do you know what your gifts are? Can you accept that there is something in particular that you are meant to do while you are here on earth? Do you need help with tapping into your power within? Can I support you as you seek your assignment?

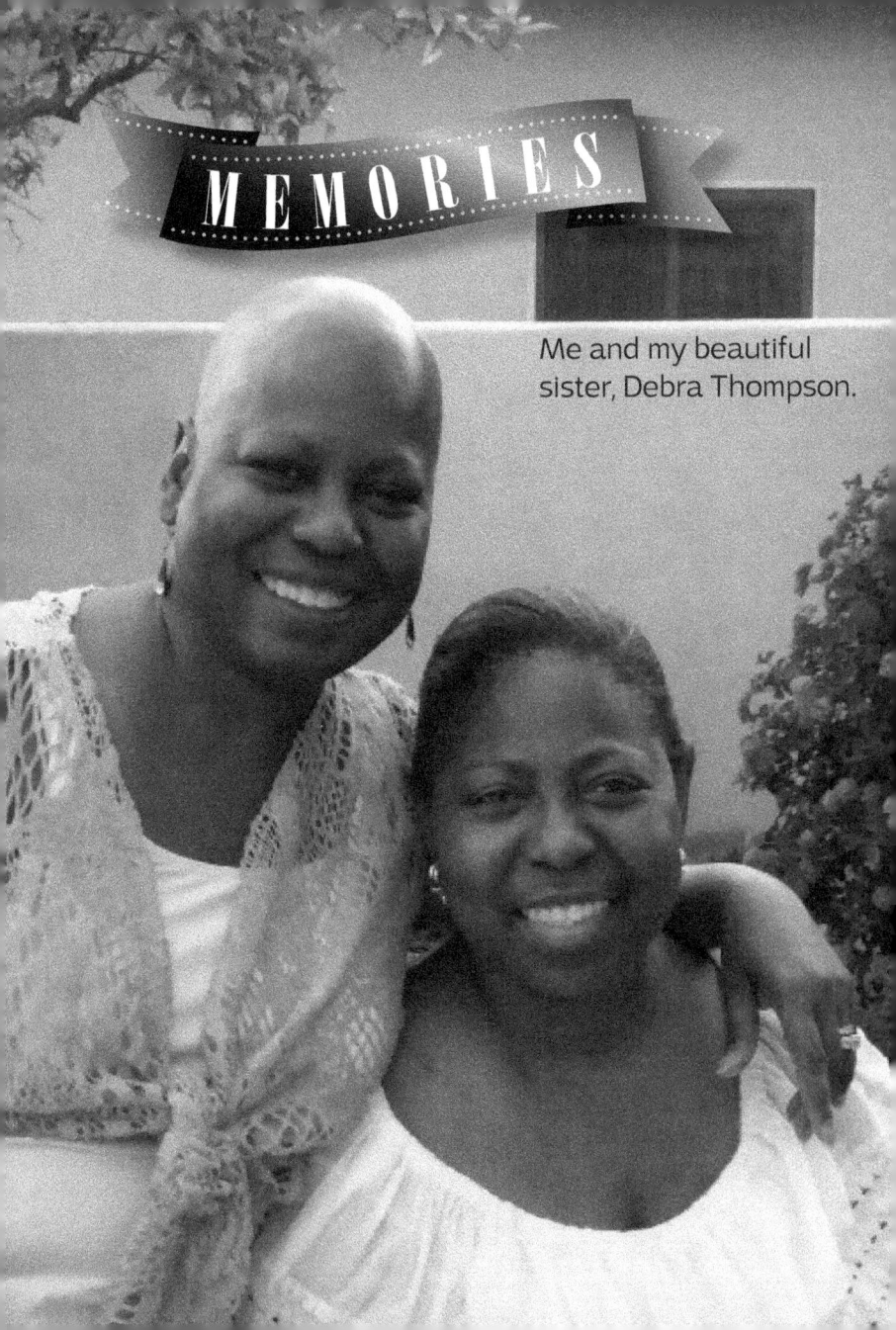

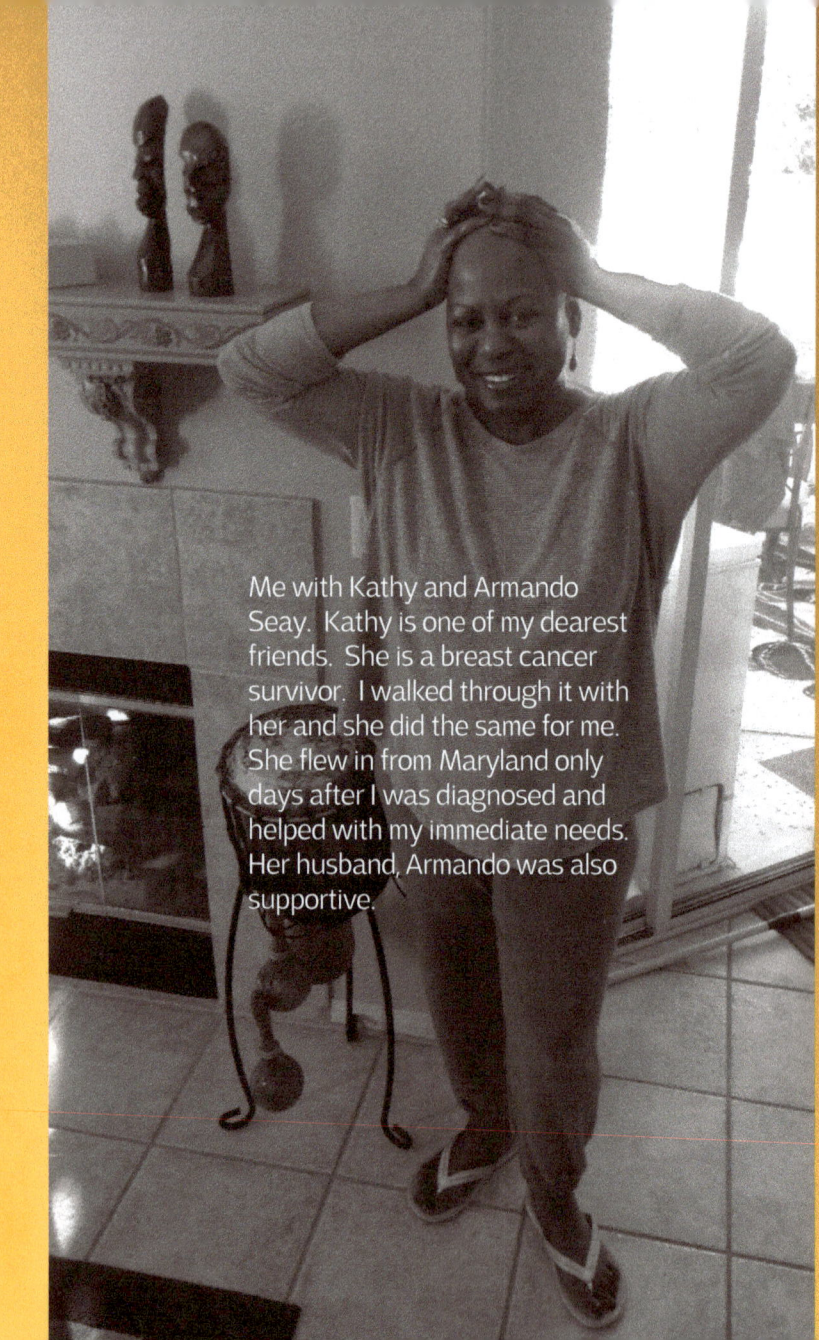

Me with Kathy and Armando Seay. Kathy is one of my dearest friends. She is a breast cancer survivor. I walked through it with her and she did the same for me. She flew in from Maryland only days after I was diagnosed and helped with my immediate needs. Her husband, Armando was also supportive.

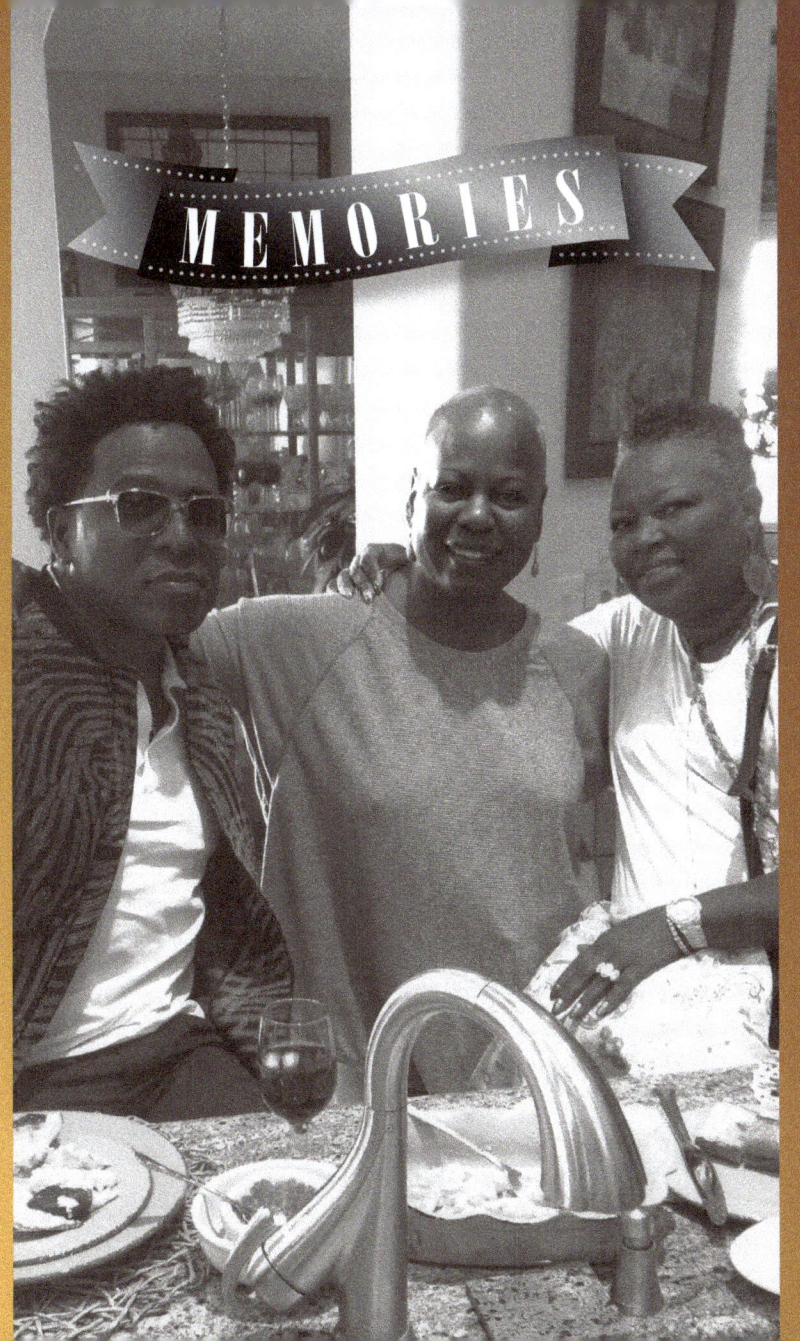

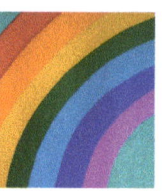

GOD'S PROMISE #5

I will provide for you.

"The Lord is my shepherd, I lack nothing."

Psalm 23:1

CHAPTER REFLECTION

Take the time now to answer a few of the questions asked of you in this chapter. What are your next steps?

CHAPTER REFLECTION

"And, God is able to bless you abundantly, so that in all things at all times, having all that you need, you will abound in every good work."

2 CORINTHIANS 9:8

CHAPTER 6
BLESSED TO BE A BLESSING

Restoration has always been a part of the master plan for my life. God did not restore me for me only. If He had, it would be the end of the story. My healing from stage III breast cancer allows me to speak light into dark places. I can now speak life where crippling fear would otherwise dominate. Simply put, I am in awe of the workings of God. For years I would be surprised by how especially good God was to me, because I knew how inconsistent I was in my relationship with him. He could turn a situation right side up in ways that baffles the most brilliant minds.

What I learned through my personal experience with God is that when He blesses you, He blesses all things concerning you. God shows up big. His authority is unmatched so that when He performs His works there could be no doubt that it was a supernatural occurrence. God can lift us out of holes and circumstances where no other option seems possible. This is the business of restoration. It seeks to change everything. It changes our lives, our finances, the trajectory of our children's lives, broken marriages are made over, dormant dreams come to life, stinking thinking turns to hope, sadness turns to joy, and chaos becomes order. This is what happens when faith the size of a mustard seed is activated for his works.

> "Behold, I make a covenant before all thy people, I will do marvels, such as have not been done in all the earth, nor in any nation . . ."
>
> Exodus 34:10

Days after leaving Exuma, Hurricane Irma tore through the Caribbean. It was August 30, 2017 and Hurricane Harvey had just hit days earlier. As a Category 4 storm off the coast of Texas, Hurricane Harvey had been described as the worse storm since Hurricane Celia in 1970. These storms displaced millions of people without food, water, and other basic items.

Stanley and I had made it back to the United States, but not home to California. We arrived in Fort Lauderdale, where we remained for days at the home of my sister, Debra, and her husband Bruce. We were unable to travel due to limited flight schedules and hundreds of cancelled flights.

While at Debra and Bruce's home, we could not help but be fixed on watching the news and feel troubled by the plight of so many people. Quietly, I asked myself what I could do to help those who needed it so desperately. I remembered how I felt watching the suffering of families in Louisiana in the aftermath of Hurricane Katrina in August 2005. Although I sent a little money to help a few families, it was always in my heart to do more. The lives of thousands would never be the same after Hurricane Katrina. Regrettably, I did not do as much as I could have done. This time would be different.

Before leaving Florida, I was able to coordinate a large delivery of rain and work boots to families in Houston, Texas. The nonprofit organization that I co-founded and serve as president has an ongoing initiative called Boots on the Ground. The International Black Women's Public Policy Institute (IBWPPI) launched this initiative to support families in rural communities a year prior to the hurricanes in Haiti, Ghana, Belize, and The

Bahamas. The goal is to collect slightly worn boots from groups such as firefighters, police officers, mechanics, labor union workers, and the public. The IBWPPI prepares them for shipment and distribution in places where natural disasters have caused flooding and devastation.

For a few days, maybe even a week, I felt good about having done something to help others that was significant; but it was not enough. A tugging in my spirit continued. I wanted to do more because the need was so great. It was not too long before the answer came to me. I had an idea that I thought my family would not be too happy about; yet, I believed they would understand.

In 2005 following the infamous Hurricane Katrina, I wanted desperately to become a chaplain for the purpose of going to New Orleans as an official spiritual counselor. During that time, it seemed that all of New Orleans needed healing and poor people were in the greatest despair.

My idea did not work out as I had hoped, and that opportunity closed. Over the years I continued to think about becoming a spiritual counselor to those living in the aftermath of a natural disaster.

Two weeks following Hurricane Harvey, I learned the Small Business Administration (SBA) was hiring hundreds of people to serve as customer service representatives. Survivors of Hurricanes Harvey and Irma would be able to secure low interest rate SBA loans to replace property loss, and repair and rebuild their homes and businesses. I applied and was quickly hired. Stanley was extremely supportive and was on standby to travel with me if I needed him. The blessing of being retired is that we could move about as freely as we wished. My greatest blessing is having a life partner who will support me even when he does not really understand.

The training was conducted over a five-day period in Sacramento, California. Following the training, I was sent to Corpus Christi, Texas along with six individuals in my class. I disclosed to a few of my classmates, during the week of training, that I had a physical limitation resulting from a major surgery just a few months earlier. I also asked for an assurance of help from one classmate I trusted with carrying my luggage and on some days, helping me get dressed.

We arrived in Corpus Christi, Texas where the SBA had set up several new disaster recovery centers. We had a few hours to get checked into the hotel and report to our assigned disaster center. We were divided into two groups of three team members. Each group had a rental car that was shared among the members of the group. We each were expected to drive. It was my blessing that there were three of us in the group, because I had not resumed driving since my surgery. I could drive, but not without some pain in my right arm. Peter and Christine, my teammates, offered to share the driving. I cooked in my room and shared meals with them from time to time. Peter thought it was a more than fair trade-off for driving. Christine and I were so nervous whenever Peter drove. He was an overly cautious driver and we all got a good laugh whenever he was behind the wheel.

Driving through the streets of Corpus Christi was a shocking experience. There was devastation all around. It seemed like a war zone, where no structure escaped the flood waters and the mighty gusts of wind. I prayed silently. I was not sure how God was going to use me in this situation however, I knew that I was prepared to be of service.

We were greeted by our team leader in the field, who was to be our direct contact for the coming weeks. Following a brief orientation and introductions to others on the team, she relieved us of our duties for the rest of the day and the following day. She sensed our astonishment and knew we needed to gather ourselves to be ready to face the survivors on Monday morning.

Christine, Peter, and I drove around to familiarize ourselves with the area. We were advised to go shopping for food and personal supplies because our time would be so limited when we began working the planned 12-hour days.

We talked with community folks we met in stores and learned what life had been like for the few weeks following the hurricanes. This gave us a glimpse of what we could expect once we were working at the disaster center. It was difficult to hear the stories that folks were eager to share with us. However, I was grateful to be available to talk through their life changing experiences.

Before we could make it back to our rooms, we received a telephone call from the regional supervisor asking if we would give up our day off and report to another disaster center nearby that really needed some help. It was a Saturday afternoon and they had lines of people needing to be helped. We agreed and quickly left to meet the team at the Corpus Christi Disaster Relief Center (DRC). The team lead was an understated gentleman who gave us a briefing and got us set up immediately. There were people waiting in long lines for help, and help is what we gave. At the end of that shift, I knew I was doing the right thing. I knew I was in the right place, at the right time.

The team lead, seeing our enthusiasm, asked if all three of us wanted to work with him for the duration of the deployment. We agreed and were reassigned the next day. The big tent setup in the parking lot of La Palmera shopping center became our workstation for two full months.

Many journeys in my life prepared and led me to this center in Corpus Christi. It was unlike anything I had imagined. Serving in some way was a given for me, but being in Corpus Christi, Texas was a big surprise for me and those who knew me. I was watching this unplanned part of my life emerge. God was expanding my territory as I had prayed, but not the way I thought He would. Coming out of cancer treatment, I had envisioned something totally different for myself, but here I was, living, working, and serving others in a place unfamiliar to me, and it was exhilarating.

One after another, families came to sit with me and told me their stories. There were times when the tears flowed from them and me. Many of the stories were about how their lives were saved from the storms and how they realized what was most important to them in those moments. Survivors would bring in their photos of what they lost. The photos were all many of them had left.

Empathy and patience worked best when meeting these families. These two necessary tools could not be taught in the five-day class. You had to have those characteristics within you. You had to be fully present when working to assist these families. The lines were long, and our patience had to be longer. I prayed for the right words and for an overflow of compassion when serving these families. My blessing is that I could be a blessing in Corpus Christi. My restoration was not just for me. My restoration was to be the tangible demonstration of what God is willing to do for His children regardless of where they are or their current circumstances.

The women who survived cancer and shared the stories that I repeated in this book, blessed me by showing me what it looked like to truly believe I would be healed. Now, I have an opportunity to share my story with those I come in contact with as they struggle to believe that their circumstances would get better. Through faith, God is able to cancel the darkness in your life. He will cut short what others intend for your demise. What you are facing now, does not have to be the end of your story. One of the gifts I would like to pass on to you is the belief that a new story for you is possible. Your new story can start right now. It requires the courage to believe.

Stanley and I moved to Atlanta, Georgia in July of 2018. We are still seeking to find a routine and the best connections for us within the community. I am looking for a church home, one where the pastor is doing more than just teaching and leading. We are looking for an inspiring community. We are looking for a place where all souls are truly welcomed, particularly those who are suffering; sometimes in silence. That was once me. I was a well-churched girl child. Most of my life was spent in the church or around church people. Yet, I suffered. I suffered from damaging self-talk. I suffered from insecurity that gnawed at me from the inside. Once I became an adult, I learned how to mask my pain. The folks in the church only saw me from the outside, while I was dying on the inside. Perhaps, this is my offering in a new church. This is the blessing I aspire to be.

We are blessed to be a blessing and no blessing is too small. Recently, since moving to Atlanta, I had my first visit to Dr. Reddy's office. She is my new oncologist. Days before my scheduled visit, I could feel my nerves beginning to grow. On the morning of the scheduled visit, I prayed while taking my shower. I was conflicted. I heard myself praying for a clear report and praying that there was no cancer present in my body. As I prayed that prayer, I asked myself, if I truly believed that I was healed. If I believed that, why was I praying for healing again?

Quickly, I shifted my prayer to thanking God for restoring my body completely. I also asked God to help me calm my nerves and to cast all my fears away by trusting in Him. I asked Him to help me keep the main thing, how blessed I am, in front of my thoughts. These few minutes changed my morning from being filled with anxiety and fear to one of peace and excitement.

When I arrived at the Atlanta Cancer Center, I walked in with a smile on my face. That smile was returned to me by the woman checking in patients. The lobby was clean and beautiful, with bright lights, giving the place a feeling of being brand new. Once I took my seat in the check-in waiting area, another nurse came out from behind the desk to inform me that she would be escorting me back to the doctor's waiting area. My smile got even bigger. This was not my experience two years ago, when I entered the cancer center for my first chemotherapy treatment.

On that day, in beautiful Rancho Mirage, when Stanley, Kelsey, Debra, and I stepped in the lobby, I felt the energy of a devastating disease that had come to steal the life and dreams from those of us sitting in the room. It was all bad. I remember the looks on the faces of patients, and the terror on the faces of family members. I remember how I had to fight within myself to not absorb or connect with what I was seeing. I asked Debra not to allow me to look or feel like what was presented to us on that day.

When the nurse checked me into the doctor's waiting area, she handed my files to yet another person who said she would be calling me in shortly. Stanley and I took our seats and began to discuss how pleasant the 15 minutes had been. As we sat there for a few minutes, another patient was brought in. She was alone and I could hear her conversation with the woman at the check-in desk. She was explaining that she had been a patient 10 years prior, but that this was a new referral. That was all I heard as her voice cracked just a bit. When she sat down across from us, I looked up to acknowledge her and saw the tears welling up in her eyes. I got up without letting Stanley know what I was getting ready to do, went over to her and offered her a hug.

This beautiful young mother of two little girls collapsed on my shoulder, weeping, and began to thank me for seeing her need. She shared with me that she was a 10-year breast cancer survivor, but unlike before, she now has two young children who need her, and she was afraid. All I had was a shoulder, hug, and a prayer. Our encounter lasted for less than seven minutes. But God! In that short time, He allowed both of us to be blessed.

I am blessed to be a blessing to others in need. There are testimonies to be shared and I have asked an incredible man to join me and share his testimony with you. I invite you to share these stories and yours, as far and wide as you can. Someone you know may need to hear one of these testimonies to encourage them. Ask God to help you reach that special person, with a unique life crisis, in need of a glimmer of hope.

TESTIMONY

Thomas W. Dortch, Jr.
Chairman Emeritus of 100 Black Men of America, Inc.
and President and CEO of TWD, Inc.

Thirty-one years ago, I found myself in the greatest battle of my life. I was confronting mortality head on. I had undergone several hours of major surgery for one of the deadliest cancers ever documented, Adenocarcinoma of the small intestine. It was a cancer that had a 92 percent mortality rate. I had lived a healthy life and never had any type of surgery prior.

Early one morning a few days after the procedure, a chaplain entered my hospital room to discuss my condition and my faith. He began the conversation by asking me if I was angry with God? I was somewhat shocked by his question. I pondered why he would he ask me such a question.

My response was emphatic. Why would I be angry with God? I sang God's praises for allowing me 38 wonderful years. My feelings were, if I did not live another hour, I thanked God for my blessings and the time I had on earth already. I was grateful, no matter what might have happened because, I knew God and I knew that God knew me. The chaplain's response was that I clearly did not need his counseling.

I am writing this testimony just a few weeks after my 60th birthday. The surgery was successful, and I have lived a healthy life 22 years after my cancer surgery. I am here today because of the blessings from God, access to excellent doctors and medical care, the love of my family, and the support of my extended family of brothers from the 100 Black Men of America.

Today, I continue to thank God for allowing me to be in the 8 percent of survivors of a deadly cancer. Since my diagnosis and treatment, I have walked my daughter down the aisle to be married. She was nine years old when I was diagnosed. I have attended my son's college graduation from Florida A&M University. He was two years old at the time of my diagnosis.

I think about how I can share my story and my blessings with young people on a daily basis, particularly those who may feel left out and left behind. God is faithful. He will never leave you or forsake you. I share my story with young people so that they would come to trust in a higher power and allow that trust and power to rule over their lives.

GOD'S PROMISE #6

I will never leave you.

"Give thanks to the Lord, for He is good;
His love endures forever."

Psalm 118:29

# CHAPTER REFLECTION

CHAPTER REFLECTION

"I am making a covenant with you. Before all your people I will do wonders never before done in any nation in all the world.

EXODUS 34:10

CHAPTER 7
WHOLE, PERFECT AND COMPLETE

This book is my seventh published offering since I began writing 20 years ago. Growing up, I never aspired to become a writer. In fact, it never occurred to me that writing for others was an option for a girl like me. I had no reason to believe that my story would be of interest to anyone outside of a few people in my immediate family.

Thinking first about this book, I had no idea that it would be about anything other than my physical health and healing from breast cancer. When Dr. Law gave me a clean bill of health, pronouncing that I was an official cancer survivor, I believed that was how I would end this story of victory. It was how I always approached a writing assignment, knowing the ending at the beginning. Once I knew the ending, I would build the rest of the story and lead the reader to the end.

In preparing for each of my previous book projects, a significant amount of time was spent on thinking about the end of each book. The ending was the message I wanted the reader to take away from the reading. Each book I have written was like having an intimate conversation with someone special to me.

Restoration: Seven Promises of God was different. The ending continued to change with each chapter I wrote. It was a bit confusing and frustrating. After a year of writing and rewriting, I decided to put the project down and simply begin to live my life as an extremely grateful survivor. It was time for me to enjoy the miracle of my life and all of my new and wonderful blessings.

Everything seemed brand new. My mornings began with prayers and meditation. The quiet time often transported me back to my childhood, growing up in The Bahamas. I remember, in 1965, at seven years old, arriving at my new home in Nassau, Bahamas, filled to the brim with childish joy and undisturbed happiness. Shortly after my arrival, I was introduced to my

Aunt Kathleen's God. She would read to me Matthew 19:14, where Jesus said, "Let the little children come to me, and do not hinder them for the kingdom of heaven belongs to such as these." Aunt Kathleen's God became my God. I learned about how He loved me and all of the children of the world. "Red and yellow, black and white we were all precious in His sight. Jesus loves the little children of the world." This scripture and song still anchor my faith today.

Through my healing process, thoughts of Aunt Kathleen's teachings brought me peace that would soothe the unsettling days and help me find my way back to my daily routines. Everything had changed. I had physical limitations to navigate. My body image would be forever different. The residual effects of the chemotherapy were memory loss and extreme fatigue that would come upon me with little to no warning.

Aunt Kathleen's God, my God, had healed me from a disease known for cutting short the lives of thousands of women, men and children. In my mind, as I began writing this book, I wanted that message to be the ending that you would read about and rejoice with me. I wanted the world to know that God was still in the healing business and that my life was the profound evidence of that fact.

What I did not know at the beginning of this book project was that God would allow my life to bear witness to much more than His power to heal us from disease. My story is a reminder that God is the maker, designer, and creator of everything about me. He alone has the power and authority to remake and restore me to the perfection that I once was. The eighteen months of writing and thinking about what I would include in this book was filled with a steady stream of metaphoric comparisons and biblical lessons. I thought long and hard about how much time I spent asking myself why I did not excel in areas I intended. Why had I not completed my PhD? Why was I not as successful as I had planned on being at 60-years-old? Why were my children not following the path I thought I designed for them to follow? All of these questions were racing through my mind while on this journey towards complete healing. I needed more than the physical healing that had already happened. All of me needed healing; my mind, body, and spirit.

There were so many questions about my life that deserved answers. Like the paralytic man at the pool in Bethesda, told in

John 5:1-9, I spent far too much time showing up, but not yet ready to receive. My subconscious belief was that I was a victim of something external. The man at the pool believed he was not healed in 38 years of showing up because without someone's help, he could never be the first person in the pool once the waters were stirred up by a healing angel. He complained that others steadily jumped in front of him. He was a comfortable victim for 38 years, until he was specifically asked by Jesus, "Do you want to be healed?" When he finally answered simply "yes", he was healed. It was the simplest question to the most complex crises in his life.

This road I am on now is different from the road I was on just two years ago. There was an important shift that took place in my life by way of a seven-month ordeal with cancer. Everything about me has changed, I have been restored by the master builder. He answered the prayer for healing that Gael T. Davis introduced to me before my first treatment in January 2017. He commanded every cell, electrical and chemical impulse, tissue, joint, ligament, organ, gland, muscle, bone, and every molecule in my body to come under complete and perfect health, strength, alignment, balance and harmony. In that same prayer, I asked God to re-create me and restore me. Guess what? He did.

He allowed me to see places and spaces where He extended grace and mercy to me repeatedly. He showed me through this journey how He never left me, even in those times when my actions were a blatant invitation for Him to get out of my life and to leave me alone. God kept His promise to me for over 50 years when He spoke to me at seven years old. I was still His little girl.

For 50 years, I stepped in and out of my relationship with God. As much as I knew He loved me and wanted the best for me, I rebelled and wanted to break free to do my own thing in my own way. Every step of the way I wanted to modify our relationship, modify the agreement that we established years before. Praise God, He knew me better than I knew myself. He knew what I really needed and made it possible for me to receive it.

I was tired of living a life mired by shame and guilt. This is how I would characterize my life as a teenager. I felt as if I had been robbed of my birthright to be happy. The adults, especially the women, insisted on cutting off my authentic loud laughter. It was not appropriate for "good girls to be heard squawking," the adult women would say. But I and a few others would do it anyway, in spite of the harsh reprimands that followed. The way I understood the environment and the norms of my

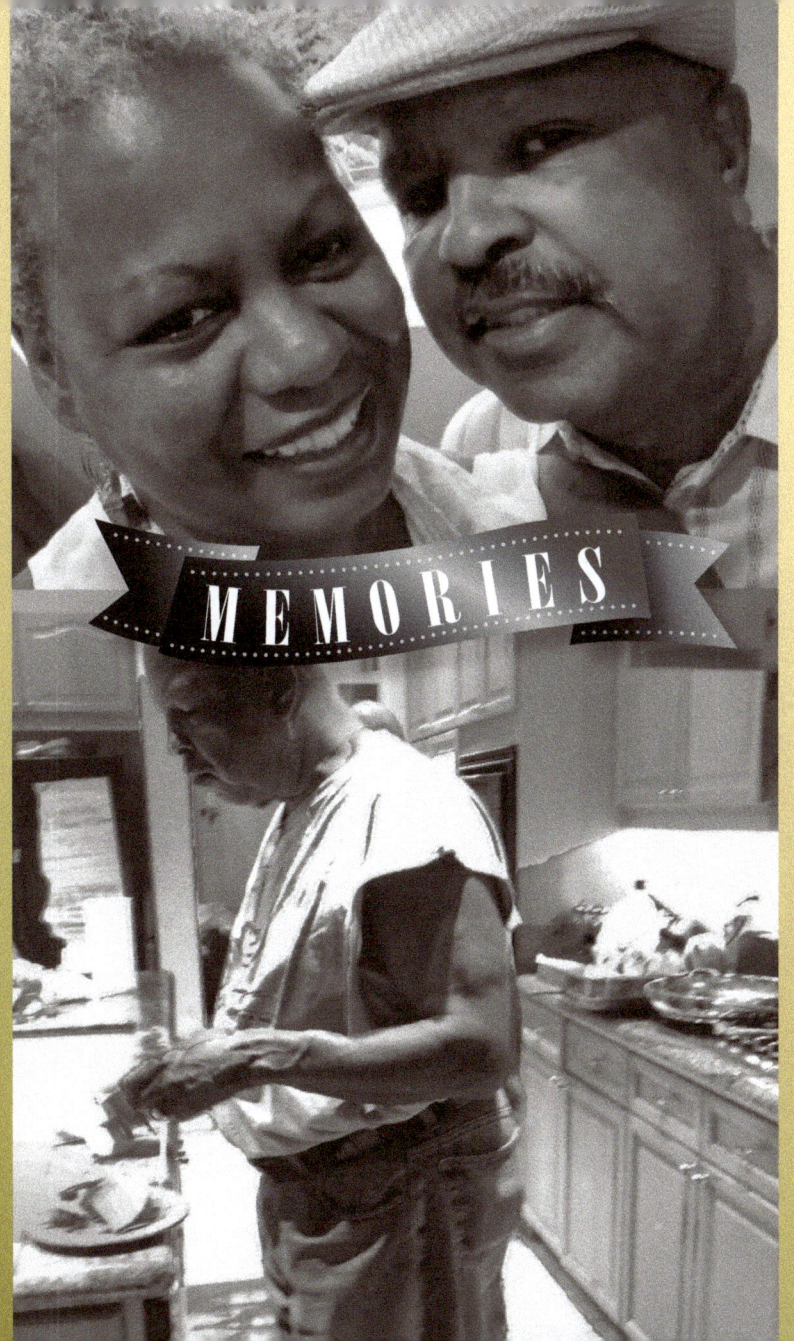

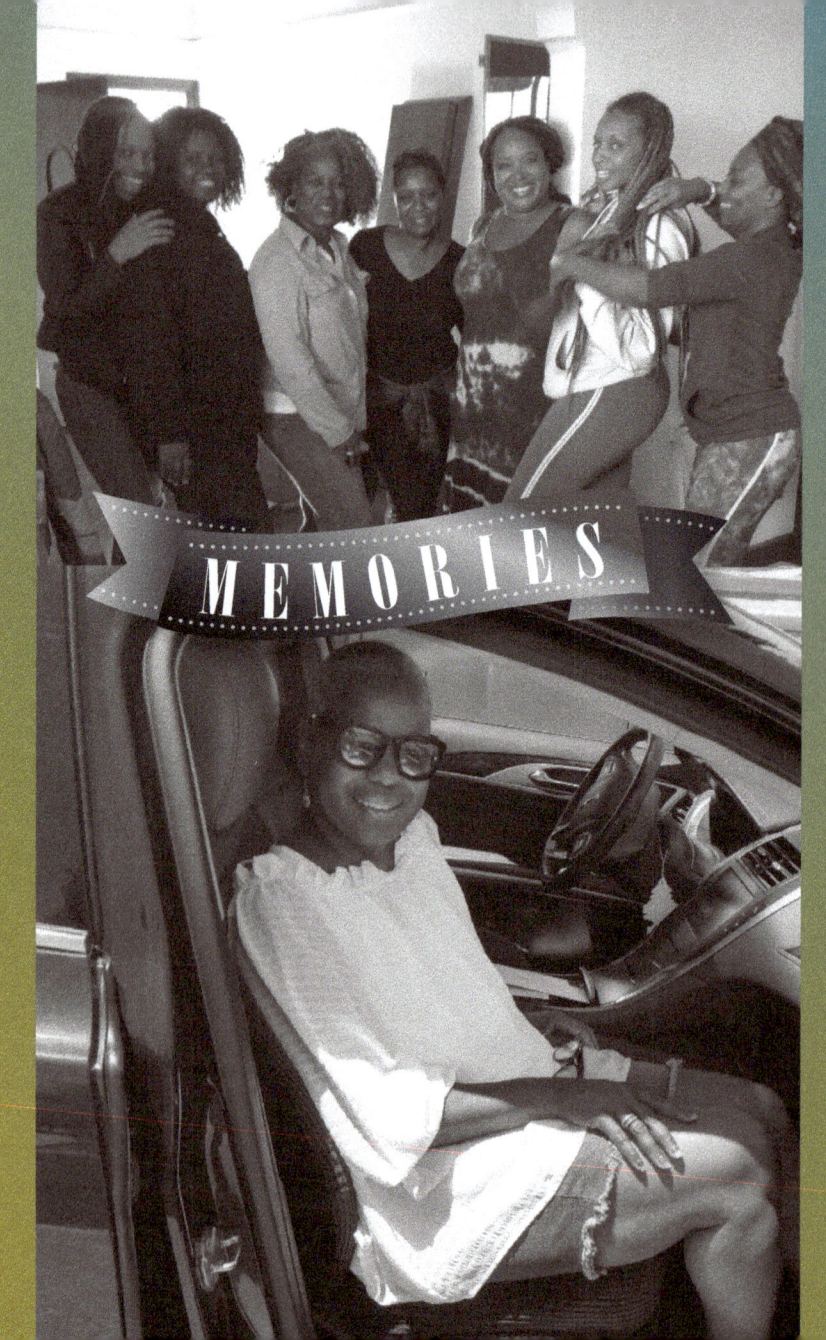

community was that nothing good came from "over the hill" (that is how my neighborhood was described). Good girls did not come from neighborhoods like mine, nor from broken, poor families like mine. The women insisted that we pretend to be good girls.

Every day, the women of "The Lily of the Valley Corner" would watch carefully for the slightest infraction I would make. No mistake went unreported to my Aunt Kathleen who was the authority on how good girls should act. I soon perfected how to pretend to be a good girl. I even participated in the training of other good girls. Forty-five years later, the weight from the mountain of guilt and shame came crashing down on me when a planned charity trip took an unexpected detour down a very painful road.

In March 2018, I led a group of women to The Bahamas for an international conference of women committed to global philanthropic work. One of the planned activities was to adopt a local library in an under-served community. We would partner with local community leaders to provide new books to the library's inventory and find other ways to establish a meaningful partnership. One of these leaders within the group, my dear friend, Cynthia Heard, spearheaded this project and worked with Delerice

Knowles-Mackey, to design and implement the vision for what we called the International Black Women's Public Policy, Reading Room Initiative-Bahamas. I had no direct involvement in the planning details and therefore, I was met with the biggest surprise of my life, on launch day, when we pulled up to the Lillian G. Weir Coakley Library building. It was renamed and dedicated to Mrs. Coakley in July 2004. This small, unkempt building was the first library I ever stepped foot into as a young girl in primary school in The Bahamas. I must have been around eight years old. Lillian Coakley was the stern librarian who worked there for 37 years. She taught me and all the other young children from that poor neighborhood how to use the library. It was a building that housed the most precious resources that were the link between our poor circumstances and success beyond our dreams.

Mrs. Lillian Coakley knew all of the children who frequently came to that library. She taught us to love books. She encouraged reading, knowing that reading would shape our ideas, and quench our thirst for knowledge. She knew me as well as she knew most of the children from the neighborhood. Her knowing me, seeing me, and believing in me, became seared in my mind as some of the most memorable parts of my life.

Mrs. Coakley stood as a character witness for me at age 16 years old after I was sexually violated, and then accused of giving consent to the thief. Although, far too many girls were victims of rape in our community, far too few of these crimes were ever reported. I was not going to allow "Leonard" the rapist, to get away with hurting me and attempting to destroy my life. Against my Aunt Kathleen's wishes, I told the police. I filed a formal complaint, and the crime was carelessly investigated and quickly dismissed as my word against Leonard and his legal team. I was left to carry that inner pain that changed my life for over four decades. Much of what happened, I buried inside so that I could carry on with my life. My emotional survival would depend on my being as far away from where this violation took place as possible. Thank God, I designed my own escape plan.

In my late twenties and early thirties, through therapy, I learned that I had displayed many of the symptoms of Abandoned Child Syndrome. For much of this time period, I felt emotionally abandoned. My first marriage at 21 years old was one of many solutions I thought would bring me peace. I needed peace from that brokenness that was a constant reminder of the lack of value that was, and is, imposed on the lives of too many poor black girls, living in the wrong neighborhoods, and who struggled to be seen, heard and believed.

I had been a student of Carolyn Keen, one of the ghost authors for the Nancy Drew series of books. This fictional girl detective solved many problems. She was unique and courageous. In my own way, I solved my big problem. I ran away from the community that perpetrated crimes against girls like me. The same community that expected us to become contributing citizens also failed us by not protecting us. It was common practice to dismiss the claims of young girls; the rape culture was alive and well in my community called "over the hill." I was not going to change it or stop it. The best that I could do was to survive it, as I did.

On that Saturday morning in March 2018, pulling up in front of what once was the Grants Town/Southern Public Library, on a bus with 30 women witnesses, another 20 plus local leaders and children from the community dressed in their beautiful red and white uniforms as I would have been 45 years ago, I realized that my 16-year-old self had not healed. What was buried deep inside of me, the painful memories, began to unearth as I saw the bronze plaque on the wall with Lillian Weir Coakley's name and the photograph of her at the entrance. I needed help from my friends on the bus who had no idea what was going on inside of me. I walked into that little building which felt like a sacred space and stood before Mrs. Coakley's picture and thanked her for helping me, for seeing me and believing in me. Tears of sadness rolled uncontrollably down my face and the faces of a few dear friends who stood beside me, not knowing what was happening.

The celebration after I shared my story for the first time was filled with such joy and shared tears. Telling my story from the podium was not the planned reading room launch message I had prepared. However, this message was a message of love, courage, determination, forgiveness, and indeed restoration. The Master Builder knew all the bandages I had put in place, over the years, over these wounds, had worn out. There would be no more repairing and patching. There would be no more bandages on these deep gaping wounds. Restoration was the only answer and my God was the only one able to deliver that solution in that very moment.

What was needed had been planted inside of me at my creation. What "Leonard" could not do was penetrate the invisible armor of protection over my life.

I am writing this chapter during Holy Week, days after Palm Sunday. This week has always held the same meaning for me. In spiritual practice, this week has been a time to reflect on sorrow and the horrific treatment of Jesus Christ by the community that He had hoped would see Him for the good that He represented. Instead this community would turn on Him and test Him to His physical death.

This is what often happens in life. We are faced with unimaginable obstacles that challenges our very existence. So often, we are simply not ready to handle these painful occurrences such as unexpected deaths, major illnesses, divorces, bankruptcy, betrayal, and failures of any kind. We find ourselves with our backs against the wall, wondering how we would possibly make it through. Then Almighty God steps in, responding to our prayers, responding to the master plan for our lives, bringing forth the courage and will to fight for the truth about ourselves.

At the memorial service for Nipsey Hussle, a popular Los Angeles rapper and philanthropist, his grieving fiancé Lauren London quoted something he had recently said to her,

"The game is going to test you, never fold, stay 10 toes down. It's not on you, it's in you. What's in you, they can't take away." That message is for everyone, regardless of age.

My God can do all things. He can fix broken hearts. God can and will remove the pain from grief and loss of life that tries to destroy or devastate you. I've felt this pain also when I became fatherless and motherless within a three-year period. This loss felt like a tree with roots exposed to the harsh elements of life. Oh, how I cried and longed for my mother's touch as I was going through cancer treatment. Who could help me get rooted again to become the strong and beautiful palm tree I was meant to be? Only God, all by Himself, can do for you what He did for me beloved. Trust him.

What's broken in your life? Can you trust that God is able to fix even your situation as He has mine? Allow me to offer this prayer for you:

Dear God,
 Maker and Ruler over all things. The one who in His image and likeness formed us in our mother's womb. God of our grandmother's mother, who heard

their hollow screams, who witnessed every bitter tear and whose name became the soothing salve to souls throughout eternity, here I am a writer, petitioner, and servant asking you to reveal your presence in the life of the person reading this book.

They may be saying:

Here I am feeling crushed, confused, and conflicted about my life. Here I am in search of a new way forward. I want a new relationship with you that is built on complete faith and trust in your authority over all things concerning my life. Forgive me God for trying to step in front of you and for thinking I could lead myself through the valleys, temptations, and evils of this world.

I confess to my failures; I acknowledge that I cannot make it without you. Today, dear God I surrender everything to you. I will sit and wait for my directions from you. Through prayer and the studying of your word. I am willing to live my life in a new way. Thank you for your healing power. Thank you for your promise to protect me from all harm and dangers. Thank you for reminding me that I am your child today and forever.

This book was written for you. It is a reminder to you that we all face challenges as we live this beautiful thing called life. Some challenges faced seem to be unbearable and even devastating. Cancer and other types of diseases are among the top of the list of challenges that can change our lives forever. However, cancer and these other diseases don't have to take over your life.

I have met so many survivors over the past few months since I began attending awareness events. Women of all ages are drawn together at these events to share their stories and to celebrate their individual, as well as collective victories in overcoming cancer. I am inspired by the community of survivors, some of whom are living their best lives. There is no doubt in my mind that this new road I am on is the beginning of my best life to come.

I have been restored. God has kept His promise to me.

"But I will restore you to health and heal your wounds, declares the Lord" because you are called an outcast, Zion for whom no one cares." Jeremiah 30:17

Are you ready to allow God to do the same for you? Ask Him, believe that He would, then allow Him to do His work by turning over whatever it is that you are facing to him.

"God is able to restore anything because He created everything."

BARBARA A. PERKINS, M.A.

He has granted us the authority to co-create with Him by way of faith and through prayer. Allow *Restoration: Seven Promises of God* to be the catalyst that supports your leap forward into that business idea that has been sitting deep inside of you. What about those dreams you have held in secret? Can they be resurrected? Only you can answer these questions. You have all that you need already. Do not allow courage to skip over you. Like footprints in the sand, where yours end, God's will begin.

Today is your new day. It is the day when you step into your new body protected by the full armor of God. You are not just the physical manifestation of God. You are the body, mind, and spirit on assignment for the Almighty God. He has recruited you for His mighty army and will be your protector from anything that seeks to harm you in any way. Can you believe that?

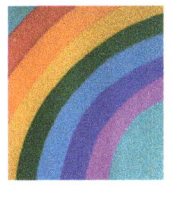

GOD'S PROMISE #7

I will protect you.

"Because he loves me," says the Lord, "I will rescue him; I will protect him, for he acknowledges my name."
Psalm 91:14

CHAPTER REFLECTION

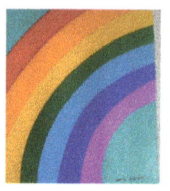

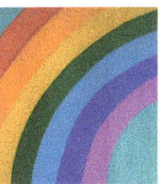

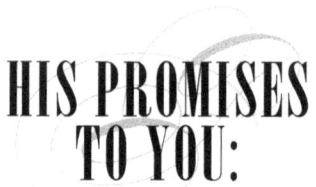

HIS PROMISES TO YOU:

1. I will be with you.
2. I will give you strength.
3. I will always love you.
4. I will give you peace.
5. I will provide for you.
6. I will never leave you.
7. I will protect you.

Maybe there are seven promises you wish to make back to God? What are they?

Use the next few pages to write them out so that you can be reminded when needed.

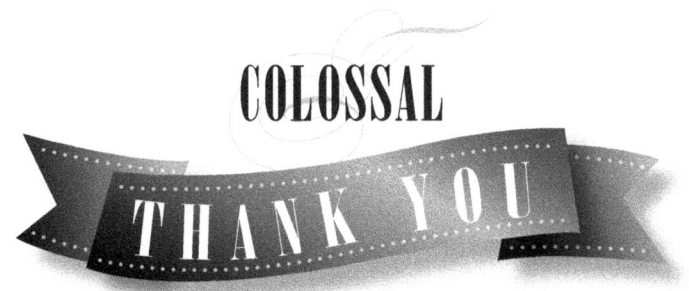

COLOSSAL THANK YOU

When someone prays for you by calling your name in their sacred time, that is a gift. When someone sends you a note or a card to let you know that they are thinking about you, while offering words of encouragement and inspiration, that too is a gift. I have been overwhelmingly gifted by others. For more than two years there has not been a day that has gone by without me being gifted a word of prayer or some special act of kindness. I did my best to hold onto every card received while going through treatment. The many bouquets of flowers received and enjoyed by me and my family make me smile just to think about them. The past two years of my life has been somewhat of a lovefest with family, friends, acquaintances, and people I do not even know. The outpouring of well wishes and prayers on my behalf has been an emotional experience.

The best I know how to do is to offer this colossal thank you to

Alicia	Candis	Denise	Gwendolyn
Allison	Carolyn	Diane	Ingrid
Almasi	Char	Drake	Iyanla
Alva	Charlene	Dwan	Jackie
Angela	Cheryl	Eartha	Jan
Angie	Chika	Ebonee	Janice
Armando	Cody	Ed	Jerry
April	Corina	Eladies	Joanne
BJ	Cortney	Eleanor	Jocelyn
Brent	Crystal	Elizabeth	Joy
Bridgit	Cynthia	Elliot	Juanita
Bernard	Darcel	Floyd	Julia
Beverly	Darrell	Francis	Kathlyn
Billie	Dawn	Gael	Kelsey
Blondell	Denae	Gladys	Kevin
Bobbie	Debra	Glenda	Khephra
Brandi	Delena	Gloria	Kim
Bruce	Delois	Gwenda	Kimberly

Laurie	Mattie	Raven	Tammilee
Lawrence	Melanie	Reena	Terry
Leah	Melinda	Regina	Thai
Leslie	Melrita	Renee	Theresa
Linda	Merilee	Rod	Tia
Lisa	Michael	Roslyn	Toni
Lois	Michelle	Ruthie	Tonya
Lori	Michellene	Sabrina	Tracey
Lula	Minga	Samantha	Tracie
Lydia	Najee	Sarah	Tyree
Maleena	Nate	Sesheida	Valarie
Marcia	Oliver	Sherman	Vanessa
Margo	Omarosa	Shingirai	Verne
Marie	Pam	Shirley	Wendy
Marilyn	Patricia	Stacie	Willa
Marsha	Paul	Stevie	Yolanda
Martha	Penelope	Susan	
Marukah	Randy	Synthia	

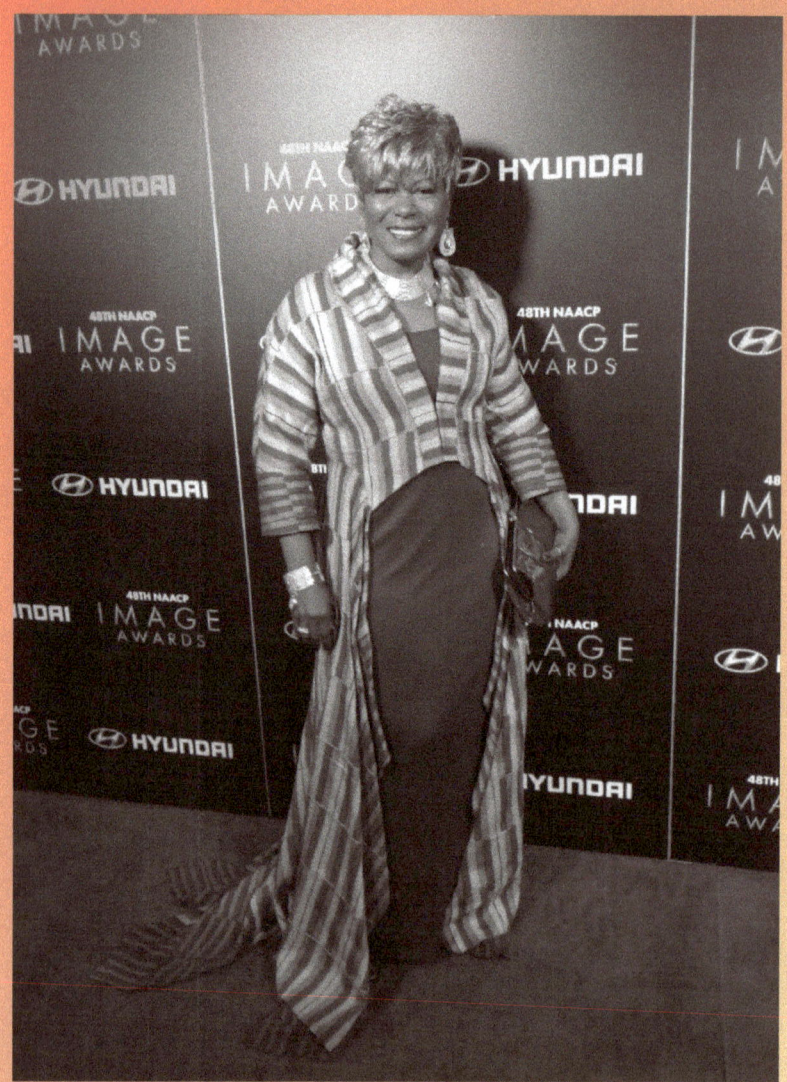

ABOUT THE AUTHOR

Barbara A. Perkins, M.A. is a certified Life Coach and ordained Minister of Spiritual Consciousness. She has been in private practice since January 2000. Her background includes leadership in higher education administration and instruction. She served for twenty-five years as a leader in nonprofit management and organizational development. Coach Barbara is a global inspirational speaker and author of six additional books.

She has been recognized nationally for her philanthropic work as well as her advocacy work on behalf of women and girls in the United States and abroad.

Barbara holds a Master of Arts degree in Human Development from Pacific Oaks College in Pasadena, California, where she served as an adjunct instructor for six years. She studied at Fielding Graduate University, in Santa Barbara, California and passed her PCC certification by the International Coaching Federation as a Life Coach. Barbara has recently moved from Los Angeles, California where she lived with her husband Stanley Perkins for 33 years. They have now retired and live in Atlanta, Georgia. They have two adult children, Kelsey and Cody Perkins, and a grandson, Emir Stanley Harrison.

Books by Barbara A. Perkins, M.A.

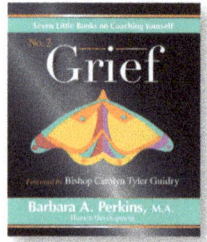
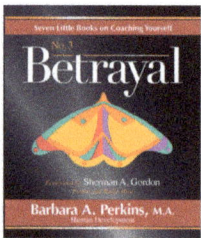
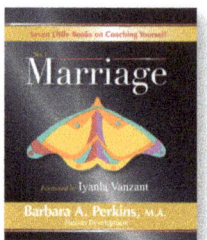
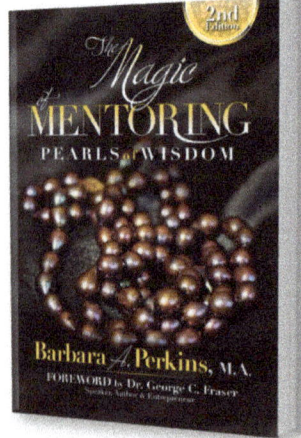
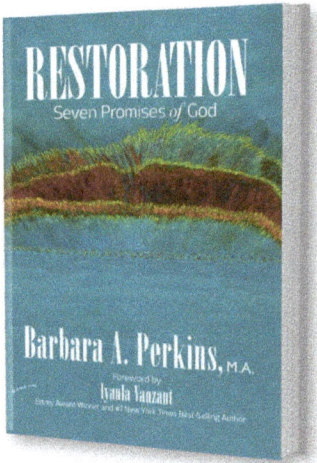

To Order Books, Visit Us At:
www.imagebuilderetc.com
www.kp-pub.com